Fasting & Anti-Inflammatory Diet for Women Over 50

Slow the Aging Process, Gain More
Energy, Experience Less Pain, and End
Fatigue by Shifting Your Eating Habits

Cristi Alonso

contained within this document, including, but not limited to, errors, omissions, or inaccuracies.

Table of Contents

"Intermittent fasting is incredibly useful in aiding fat loss, preventing cancer, building muscle, and increasing resilience. Done correctly, it's one of the most painless high-impact ways to live longer." —Dave Asprey

Introduction

Diabetes, heart disease, osteoporosis, bladder issues, cancer, depression, chronic pain, and dementia… Nine out of 10 older adults develop serious illnesses as they age, many having more than one (Nazario, 2020). If this is what "old" promises are, it's no surprise why many women fear the big 5-0.

Is it possible to bypass these health issues in your 50s and beyond? While it's impossible to give a definitive yes or no, I can say that you can take essential steps to significantly reduce your risk of serious illness as you age. Not only is it possible to be your healthiest, but also possible to feel more energized, stronger, and confident as you embrace adding another year to your life.

You might not be feeling this right now. Fatigue may set in after the smallest tasks. Is this how the rest of your years are going to feel? Are you feeling exhausted, unmotivated, weak? No matter how much sleep you get, you still feel tired, like you haven't slept in days.

Suddenly you have more aches and pains. With each new birthday, there appears to be a new hindrance your body endures. Getting around is a chore in itself. The fatigue and pain are taking away your confidence as going about your daily routine are more challenging.

You're just shy of 50. Or maybe you've made it past this milestone, but you fear that in a few years, you'll be relying heavily on others to take care of you.

And let's not ignore the biggest frustration. As you gain another year in age, you seem to gain a few more pounds around the waist. You've tried every diet you've come across, but nothing seems to get rid of that stubborn belly fat. As much as you fight your cravings for sweets and carbs, you can't resist, so you give in. You may have never struggled with your weight before, or you could easily drop those extra pounds quickly. But now, the more you try to get back to a healthy weight, the more weight you seem to gain.

Is this all just a part of getting old? You may be telling yourself this to make sense of what's going on with your body because you simply can't find another explanation. Many women fall into this trap. They believe they just have to accept the changes their bodies are going through, and there's nothing that can be done.

This doesn't have to be your excuse anymore. You don't have to just shrug it off and convince yourself that old age just brings on all these ailments, and there's nothing you can do about it. You also shouldn't think that you'll just get medication to ease the discomfort from the pain and health issues you encounter.

There's a better way. A much better way! One that doesn't rely on prescriptions. Or living a life through restrictions advised by the health care profession that tells you to play it extra safe, so you don't injure yourself or because your health is too poor to endure all the fun things you used to live for.

That's no way to live, and you don't have to accept it as your future.

If you have a robust immune system, you can avoid many diseases and the usual strife that getting older brings. One of the best ways to enhance your 50s and beyond is through a balanced lifestyle that promotes a healthy gut, fights inflammation, and protects against many conditions that put you at a greater risk as you get older. A balanced lifestyle encourages the right diet, eating approach, physical activity, sleep, and stress management. While this seems like a lot to change all at once, each of these healthy habits only requires small efforts and minimal changes.

As I approached 50, I struggled to maintain my weight, had unexplained muscle and joint pain, and constantly felt unwell. Despite overcoming several minor illnesses, I never regained my stamina and strength. I never felt 100% well and often felt weaker and less healthy than before.

I began to wonder how I would feel in the coming years and asked myself, "Would I be able to live a satisfying and enjoyable life, or would my health continue to decline?"

I felt somewhat discouraged about my future, thinking there was nothing I could do to improve my situation. I thought it was just a part of aging, so I reluctantly accepted it. I thought managing any pain, fatigue, and health conditions could mean relying heavily on medication, which would only further lower my quality of life and didn't feel like an option.

However, I remember a time when I was extremely sick and could hardly get out of bed. When I finally recovered from the virus, it took all my energy just to stand up. I knew this was not the life I wanted, so I made a decision to find a better way.

I was astounded that some women in their 70s could keep up with 30-year-olds, and I was determined to take control of my health and find positive solutions to these challenges. With a proactive mindset, I was confident that I would continue to lead a fulfilling and vibrant life, despite any setbacks along the way.

I reached out to a close friend who was a natural health practitioner for help, and with her guidance, I started making gradual changes to my lifestyle that made me feel healthier. I took the information and advice my friend provided and did my own research to find more ways to improve my health. It was a long journey, but I finally found a healthy, maintainable lifestyle. I want to spare you months or years of searching for the right approach to your health and wellness.

I wrote this book to encourage you to take control of your health. To begin making simple changes that can have a profound impact on your health and happiness. Whether you're near 50 or over, the information in this book will change the course of the rest of your life.

I know what it's like to suffer from pain and low energy, relying on others to help you get through the day. I don't want to depend on my family and burden them with my poor health. I want to squeeze a few more decades out of this life, and I want to do it full of energy and vitality. I don't fear getting older or dread what another year brings because I have learned a holistic approach to maintaining optimal health.

I want to inspire other women to take control of their life at any age. I want you to feel the energy you once had. To move with ease and without pain. I know this is possible as I have experienced this and more.

Through this book, you will learn effective ways to combat the most common ailments for women over 50. You'll learn the best ways to improve your health, reduce inflammation, and manage your weight without a strict diet plan. You won't just learn what to eat but when to eat, so that your body begins to work with you to burn away stored fat and increase your energy level.

Finally, you'll learn how to fall in love with exercise while discovering the most effective types of physical activity to help keep you strong and flexible. I hope that by the end of this book, you'll feel more confident and ready to embrace your golden years. I hope that you take the small steps to live out the rest of your days with excitement and adventure. Because it's possible. If you're ready to feel younger and more vibrant, let's get started with the most important factor that can either cause you to feel sick and tired or more vibrant and energized.

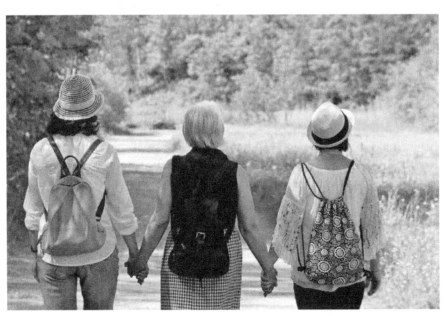

Chapter 1:

How Food Impacts Your Health

"Let food be thy medicine and medicine be thy food."—Hippocrates

The start to a healthy life begins with what you eat. This isn't new and profound knowledge. You're already aware that eating the right foods leads to weight loss, but what you eat has a more significant impact on your overall health than just your weight. Understanding how food impacts your health will help you make the best food choices to improve your health as you get older. You'll learn that food can be your best form of medicine, or it can introduce and promote a decline in health. This connection runs beyond your waistline, and it's one of the root causes of inflammation that further damages your internal processes. Eating the right whole foods provides your body with what it needs to perform optimally at any age.

Impact of Food on Your Health

Most of us know that we need food to survive, but we don't know the role food plays in our health, and it connects to our overall satisfaction in life. From a young age, we learn that we should eat our vegetables and that sweets are bad, yet we choose to eat highly processed foods that are quick to make or pick up at a drive-thru.

Have you ever considered why those vegetables are so much better? Why should sugar be avoided? Or, how those convenient foods are damaging your health? While we know what we should eat, we don't know **why.**

We often look at food as a source of calories, which it is. But food is more than just calories consumed.

What Does Food Do in Our Bodies?

Food supplies our bodies with various vitamins, minerals, and nutrients. Some foods have a bountiful amount of these essential items, while others have a minimal amount. The ability of our body to function correctly relies heavily on the right balance of nutrients.

An adequate combination of nutrients is integral to how our body functions. When we lack the essential nutrients our body needs, it can't perform as it should for our best health. Going for prolonged periods without the vital nutrients our body needs leads to a decline in health.

A simplified way to understand the complex role food plays in our body is that it gives specific instructions for how our body operates. Some nutrients activate hormonal production. Others aid in cell growth and repair. Some initiate fat storage, and others trigger fat burning.

A more thorough understanding of how food functions in the body, how the body utilizes the nutrients, and the critical role food plays in proper functioning will give you a new perspective on food. One that doesn't just say you should eat more vegetables but one that also guides you to choose more nutritious foods so your body functions optimally well into your 50s and beyond.

The Connection Between Food and Disease

One of the leading causes of death in the United States is heart disease (Elflein, 2022). It is the No. 1 killer for women, followed by cancer and stroke. Heart disease can have many contributing causes, such as high blood pressure, high cholesterol, diabetes, and other questionable lifestyle choices, like a lack of exercise and smoking.

What does this have to do with the food we eat? Everything.

The foods we consume influence our blood pressure, cholesterol, blood sugar, and other body processes that keep our hearts functioning.

Unhealthy fats, like saturated fats, are in fried foods, processed oils, processed meats, and prepackaged foods. These saturated fats increase the low-density lipoprotein (LDL) cholesterol, which is the bad cholesterol in our bodies. It accumulates as plaque on the heart's artery walls. Over time, it prevents proper blood flow to and from the heart, creating the perfect storm for a heart attack or stroke.

High blood pressure exists when your blood presses against the walls of your arteries with too much force. It means your heart is working overtime to push blood to the rest of the body, and it doesn't take enough time to recover from this activity between beats. Over time, high blood pressure begins to damage the arteries in the heart. The damage creates the ideal place for plaque (LDL cholesterol) to accumulate as it begins to fill in all the little tears along the artery walls.

The main contributing factors to high blood pressure are diabetes and obesity. And what is the leading cause of diabetes and obesity? Our diet. The connection between the foods we eat and our health is closely and continuously studied. The idea of functional medicine arises from this connection.

Functional medicine looks at how diet can hinder or promote health. It examines the role that nutrients, or the lack of them, from our diets play in developing chronic conditions through their impact on the major systems in the body. The digestive tract, immune system, and detoxification systems (made up of the liver and kidneys) all play vital roles in proper health. When one of these systems begins to function poorly, overall health begins to decline.

Most of these systems reside in the digestive tract, highlighting the importance of proper nutrition for proper body functioning. Early detection of a poorly functioning system can help prevent more serious health conditions. However, this is often not enough to persuade individuals to change their diets for optimal health.

Many have a negative outlook on what it means to eat a healthy diet. There's a belief that a healthy diet means we must stick with boring, flavorless, and bland salads, giving up our favorite foods. To counter that belief, we need to rewire how we think and look at food, so we can enjoy what we eat while improving our health.

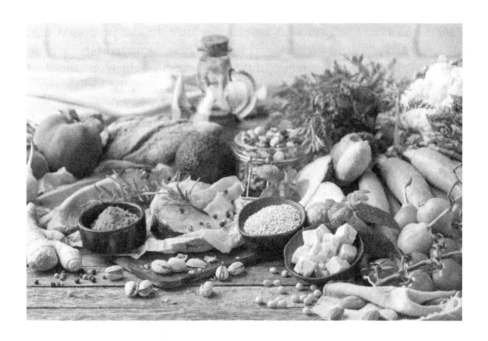

Why You Should Eat Whole Foods

Eating whole foods cleans up your diet. You eliminate nutrient-sparse foods and include more nutrient-rich foods. You may think that eating whole foods is just another dieting trap that imposes strict guidelines and rules. This misconception keeps many from giving the whole foods approach to eating a chance.

However, whole foods simplify eating a better-for-you diet and can be sustained long-term with little to no adverse effects.

What Is a Whole Food Diet?

Whole foods refer to unprocessed foods consumed as close to their natural state as possible. They do not contain artificial ingredients, unhealthy fats, refined grains, or sugars. You may have heard this referred to as clean eating. A whole foods diet is about cleaning up what you eat to experience better health, more energy, and increased vitality.

Whole Foods Versus Processed Foods

Processed foods undergo various processes that essentially strip them of the beneficial nutrients the body needs. Most people consume a diet mainly of processed foods, at least to some degree. These processed foods are things that have been pre-cooked, canned, packaged, or have nutrients added to them. If we look even closer at the term "processed," we can add many more food items to the list. Pre-cut vegetables, like bagged salads or even sliced lettuce, can be considered processed. Roasted nuts and brown rice go through a process, whether roasting the nuts or drying the rice grains.

Many foods are "processed" that still provide nutrients. When we speak of processed foods, those that can be damaging to your health are the ones that add ingredients or go through chemical processes that we want to avoid. For example, yogurt goes through a fermentation process. It is high in protein and beneficial bacteria that keep the gut healthy. It's when sweeteners, artificial flavors, and other artificial ingredients are added that the yogurt becomes less healthy.

We want to avoid highly processed foods that alter entirely the nutritional impact these foods should have. Fried foods and prepackaged meals are two of the most common processed foods consumed as a considerable portion of one's diet. However, foods containing high amounts of sugar, salt, or various ingredients we can't pronounce are typically highly processed.

Most people incorporate an abundance of these types of food, which contributes to declining health.

While some processed foods have added nutrients, it doesn't change the fact they're still highly processed. The body doesn't absorb these nutrients as thoroughly as it would if they came from organic sources. Many diet foods claiming to be low-fat or low-carb tend to have excess sodium or sugar added to them.

Whole foods are much easier to identify; you often don't have to guess whether you're purchasing something healthy. Whole foods are simple foods: fruits, vegetables, whole grains, and lean meats. They don't have an ingredient list a mile long because they're either in raw form or contain only other natural ingredients. For instance, almond butter contains raw ground almonds; some might add cinnamon, pure maple syrup, and sea salt. All the ingredients are natural and ones you recognize.

Health Benefits of Whole Food Diet

The main benefit of a whole foods diet is that foods maintain their natural nutrients. The fiber, phytochemical, and other nutrients aren't removed or destroyed during an extensive process method, as is the case with most other highly processed foods. Whole foods are nutrient-rich and fresh.

Studies have shown that a diet of whole foods helps prevent chronic diseases like cardiovascular disease. Because this way focuses on ingesting more plant-based foods, you get a variety and well-balanced intake of nutrients to allow the body to function properly.

Those suffering from health conditions, like type 2 diabetes, autoimmune disease, and heart disease, among others, can manage their symptoms by eating a whole foods diet. It provides the body with essential nutrients to keep the immune system operating correctly. It limits the intake of foods known to trigger inflammation, which causes the immune system to become overworked and out of sync.

A whole foods diet encourages eating plenty of fruits, vegetables, and whole grains, which are lower in calories. You eat significantly more on a whole foods diet than a traditional American or Western diet. For example, the average American dinner of a cheeseburger, fries, and a soft drink can add up to around 1,000 calories. A typical whole foods dinner with primarily steamed or roasted vegetables, a small lean piece of meat, and a side of whole grains is around 400 calories.

Risk of a Whole-Food Diet

Unlike other traditional diet plans, you don't necessarily need to concern yourself with calorie intake. If you shift your focus to eating more vegetables and whole grains, which are often lower in calories, there's little concern about overeating or consuming more calories than you burn. However, counting calories is a concern when you're trying to lose weight. A whole foods eating plan makes it easy to reduce your calorie intake without much tracking or stress.

However, there's a risk that when you're at a healthy weight, you may not be consuming enough calories to fuel your body. Understanding how to incorporate healthy, high-calorie foods, like avocado, nuts, dried fruits, and soy, can help you meet your necessary calorie intake while still choosing plant-based, health-boosting alternatives.

Another thing to mention is that the whole food diet shouldn't be approached as a quick-fix diet trend; many will naturally fall into a fad dieting mindset. Those who may struggle with some variation of disordered eating (binge eating, bulimia, etc.) become more hyper focused on the foods they consume. A whole foods diet simplifies eating a balanced, nutrient-rich diet, but this doesn't mean some may not still obsess, worry, or feel shame about eating foods that aren't considered whole foods.

I always encourage anyone who has struggled with yo-yo dieting or felt out of control with food to consult their primary care physician, nutritionist, or dietician to discuss their current and past eating habits.

It'll be hard to stick with a healthy diet, no matter what type you choose, if you look negatively at food, feel shame, or experience guilt about eating. It's best to repair your relationship with food and yourself first.

Whole Foods Food List

Whole foods are simple. They haven't been harshly processed. Preservatives have not been added, and there are no artificial ingredients to make the food look more appealing. Whole foods are the most beneficial because they contain the highest amounts of vitamins, minerals, and nutrients to promote good health. Many whole foods you can find at your local grocery store are mentioned below:

Grass-fed meats

- Beef

- Goat

- Venison

- Lamb

- Bison

This includes your dairy products. Milk, cheese, butter, yogurt, and ice cream should all come from grass-fed animals (cows, goats, sheep).

Free-range organic poultry

- Chicken

- Turkey

- Duck

- Quail

- Eggs

Wild caught seafood

- Fatty fish (salmon, anchovies, bass, sardines, carp, herring, mackerel)

- Lean fish (tuna, tilapia, halibut, mahi mahi, cod, trout, catfish, haddock, snapper)

- Shrimp

- Oysters

- Lobster

- Crab

- Scallops

- Squid

Plant-based proteins

- Beans

- Legumes

- Lentils

- Edamame

- Tofu

- Quinoa

- Buckwheat

- Nutritional yeast

- Pea protein

Gluten-free grains

- Oats

- Quinoa

- Buckwheat

- Teff

- Amaranth

- Sorghum

- Corn

Other whole-grains

- Wheat

- Barley

Organic natural sweeteners

- Dates and date paste

- Pure maple syrup

- Raw sugar

- Agave

- Honey

- Coconut sugar

- Monk fruit

Starchy vegetables

- Sweet potatoes

- Yucca

- Corn

- Peas

- Beans

- Legumes

- Lentils

- Squash (acorn, butternut)

Non-starchy vegetables and fruits (with high traces of micronutrients but no calories and macronutrients):

- Leafy greens (spinach, kale, bok choy)

- Cruciferous vegetables (broccoli, cauliflower, Brussel sprouts)

- Cucumbers

- Green beans

- Celery

- Mushrooms

- Beets

- Onions

- Carrots

- Artichokes

- Berries (blackberry, blueberries, strawberries)

- Melons (watermelon, honeydew, cantaloupe)

- Sea vegetables (seaweed, algae, kelp)

- Lemons

- Limes

- Herbs

Fruits

- All varieties that are organically grown, including dried and frozen fruits.

Healthy fats

- Avocados and avocado oil

- Extra virgin olive oil

- Nuts (include nut butter like cashew or almond butter)

- Seeds (chia, pumpkin, sunflower, flax. including seed oils like sesame oil)

- Coconut and coconut oils

- Tahini

- Cacao

Dairy alternatives

- Plant-based milk (almond, cashew, oat, hemp, coconut, rice milk)

- Soy-based dairy (soy yogurt, soy milk)

- Vegan cheeses (cashew cheese sauce, nutritional yeast)

What Not to Eat

What not to eat is a short list, and you're probably aware you should limit or eliminate the consumption of these items: refined or artificial sweeteners, processed meats, sugar treats and desserts, packaged foods or snacks, soda, other sweetened beverages, and alcohol. These foods provide very few nutrients and are full of empty calories.

Why Balance Is Important

Eating a balanced diet is one of the first things often recommended to those who want to improve their health, lose weight, and prevent or manage chronic disease. What does eating a balanced diet mean, though? Many may think of the "My Plate" or outdated food pyramid and think they need to eat according to these diagrams. While diagrams may serve as a starting point for understanding a balanced diet, they don't give you a clear definition of what that consists of.

A balanced diet is one that provides your body with adequate nutrition for optimal health and functionality. Nutrients come from a combination of:

- Fruits

- Vegetables

- Whole grains

- Lean protein

- Legumes

- Nuts and seeds

But, nutrients are only a part of the equation. A balanced diet also ensures you consume enough calories to fuel your body. Calories aren't the enemy, as many believe. Calories give your body energy so you can think clearly, walk, breathe, and even sleep soundly.

The number of calories you need daily will depend on your age, sex, and current physical activity level. Women who are over 50 with a more sedentary life, where they aren't physically active daily, only need between 1,600 to 1,800 calories a day. More active women will need to consume slightly more calories, between 2,000 to 2,200.

How to Achieve Balance

You want to have the right amounts of macro and micronutrients. Macronutrients consist of carbohydrates, fat, and protein. We need these nutrients in high quantities, which need to be of better quality. For instance, store-bought or pre-packaged cupcakes are a significant source of carbohydrates and fats, but these are simple carbs and saturated fats. A bowl of oatmeal with sliced banana and some coconut oil is also high in carbs, but these are complex carbs that are much more beneficial to the body than simple carbs. These need to be consumed daily as the body uses carbs, fat, and protein to fuel the functions of the body.

Micronutrients consist of all the other vitamins and minerals the body needs. There are 13 essential vitamins we should be getting in small to moderate quantities daily, like B vitamins and vitamins A, C, E, and K. These vitamins are vital for keeping the whole body functioning properly. The body needs many minerals, like magnesium, iron, sodium, and zinc, to perform certain functions. We don't need to consume all the essential vitamins and minerals daily as many of these can be stored and used later in the body.

Eating the right balance of foods guarantees we're getting the right amount of macro and micronutrients. Some simple tips to keep in mind that will help you stick to a more balanced meal plan include:

- Half of your plate should be filled with vegetables or fruit.

- A quarter of your plate should be whole grains.

- The remaining quarter of your plate should consist of lean proteins or plant-based protein sources.

- You can use dairy sparingly; consider it as a condiment or small side dish.

A balanced diet is easy to achieve. By adding more fruits and vegetables to your meals and choosing your grains carefully, you can give your body the right types of nutrients at any age!

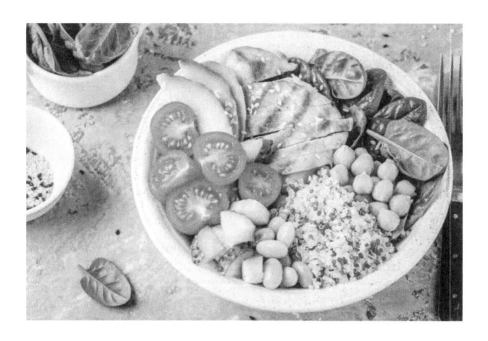

How Body Systems Work Synergistically with Others

The body consists of cells, organs, and blood vessels neatly organized into 10 different systems. Each system is responsible for maintaining the inner workings of specific parts or areas of the body. For example, the nervous system keeps the nerves working properly, and the endocrine system is responsible for hormone production and distribution. The immune system is responsible for warding off infection and keeping the rest of the body safe.

Each system is interconnected and dependent on one another to fulfill its purposes. Some systems send signals to perform specific actions. For instance, the nervous system triggers the brain to speed up your heart rate when you feel anxious. Other systems are responsible for distributing nutrients to the appropriate place to keep cells and vessels strong. The digestive tract, for example, sends plenty of calcium and iron to the skeletal system so our bones grow strong.

If one system fails to perform its job, the other systems eventually begin to decline in functionality. Even systems that seem to have no direct connections rely on one another. For instance, the skeletal system relies on the urinary tract system to remove waste produced by the bone cells. Your bones create new blood cells, which are essential for the circulatory system to deliver oxygen adequately throughout the body. This is why we look at a balanced diet and eating healthy as more than just a way to lose weight or reduce the risk of certain chronic conditions. We need to look at our diet as a complete body health approach, one that ensures all body systems are getting what they need to continue working together flawlessly.

You know there are many nutrients your body needs. You can begin to take the steps to positively impact your health by adopting a balanced diet that allows you to consume what your body needs. But what if you take this information and level it up to optimize the beneficial impact of these nutrients on your health? This is where nutrient and food synergy comes into play!

Benefits of Nutrient Synergy

Certain nutrients enhance the effects of another. When these nutrients work together, they provide more significant benefits than if you consumed them independently. Some of the physical and psychological benefits of nutrient synergy include:

- Lowering the risk of heart disease

- Reducing the risk of stroke

- Helping manage osteoporosis

- Increasing energy level

- Improving immune systems

- Improving focus and cognitive functioning

Some of the best nutrient combinations to strive for include:

- Vitamin C and iron

- Vitamins B6 and B12 with folate

- Calcium, vitamin V and vitamin K

- Vitamins C and E

- Potassium, magnesium, and calcium

Food Synergy

Food synergy is similar in concept to nutrient synergy. Certain foods can be eaten together to boost the benefits of each food. When you eat specific ingredients together, the body can more easily absorb the nutrients and use them most effectively.

Foods that should be eaten together

- Probiotics and prebiotics are like bananas and yogurt. The banana acts as a prebiotic, which helps feed the good bacteria in the digestive tract. Yogurt is a probiotic which helps introduce good healthy bacteria to the digestive tract. Eating these together helps promote beneficial bacteria growth and immediately supplies food for the good bacteria to thrive.

- Avocados or extra-virgin olive oil and fresh fruits or vegetables go well together. For example, you can combine freshly squeezed lemon juice and extra-virgin olive oil to make a citrus dressing for your salads. Fruits and vegetables have a variety of nutrients that aren't easily released when you eat them. The compounds in healthy fats, like avocados and oils, make it easier for the body to absorb certain nutrients, such as vitamins A, E, and K. They also help the body take in alpha and beta carotene, lutein, and lycopene. These further boost eye, skin, and cardiovascular health.

- Broccoli and tomatoes both have powerful cancer-preventing properties. When steamed, these properties are further enhanced. Tomatoes are also rich in the antioxidant lycopene, which promotes heart health. Broccoli has high amounts of the phytonutrient sulforaphane, which helps remove free radicals in the body and can slow the growth of tumor cells.

- Turmeric and black pepper work together to help fight cancer. Turmeric has high amounts of the powerful antioxidant curcumin. Curcumin is widely known for its anti-cancer and anti-inflammatory properties. Black pepper has a unique compound—piperine. Piperine boosts the cancer-fighting properties in the turmeric and increases the rate of absorption 1,000 times (Agarwal, 2020).

- Lemon and green tea, when consumed together, can help further boost the immune system, prevent premature aging, and combat certain types of cancer. Lemons are a significant source of vitamin C. Green tea is rich in antioxidant catechins. The power of the antioxidants in green tea is enhanced nearly 10 times when paired with the vitamin C in the lemons (Agarwal, 2020).

Now that you understand how food will enhance your health as you age, we're going to focus on what foods will lead to more success in a healthy lifestyle. Some of the misunderstood foods you should be including in your healthy diet are oils and fats.

Chapter 2:

Oils—the Good and the Bad

Many of the foods we eat, even lettuce, contain fats. Fats and oils have carried around a bad reputation for decades. Even with evidence showing that the body needs fats to function and perform certain tasks, we tend to cut out fats when trying to lose weight. Fats, however, can boost weight loss if you add the right kinds of fats to your diet.

Certain foods, like margarine, particularly the hard stick kinds, are worse for your heart than butter because they contain higher amounts of trans fat. While you certainly want to eliminate these trans-fat foods, other fats and oils are incredibly beneficial for your health, especially as you age.

What Oils Are

Oils are fats found in various plants and fish. While oils aren't a food group of their own, they provide us with nutrients like vitamin E and are essential for assisting the body in absorbing other key nutrients.

Natural oils maintain a liquid state at room temperature. Processed oils will solidify. Natural sources of oils include:

- Nuts
- Olives
- Fish
- Avocados

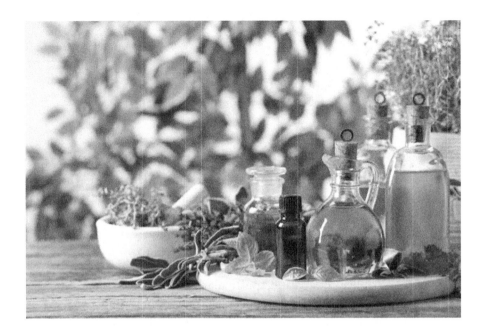

Types of Oils

You have plenty of oils to choose from—flaxseed, olive, coconut, corn, and others. Each type of oil has its own characteristics and provides varying amounts of different kinds of saturated or unsaturated fats. Some oils are better for cooking; others are best for dressing or dipping sauces. Many believe some oils are beneficial to their health, but that may not be true. Let's discuss the most common oils you probably have in your kitchen or have used because they're said to be better for your health.

Olive Oil

Olive oil contains oleic acid, linoleic acid, and palmitic acid. These are long-chain fatty acids that have been shown to reduce the risk of cardiovascular disease.

When you shop for olive oil, you may notice three different types, extra-virgin olive oil (EVOO), virgin olive oil, and olive oil. These labels give you an indication of the health benefits of the oil.

EVOO is the purest type of olive oil and contains a high level of antioxidants and vitamin E. However, once you heat the oil, it loses most of these nutrients. EVOO shouldn't be used for cooking purposes. Instead, this oil should be used for dressings, sauces, and other purposes where it will not be heated.

Virgin olive oil is a lighter, more versatile option for cooking than extra-virgin olive oil. It has a milder flavor, making it better suited to dishes that require longer cooking times or higher temperatures. Additionally, virgin olive oil goes through several processes to remove unwanted odors. The oil is also often mixed with plain olive oil to create a blend with more mild flavors and greater versatility.

Plain olive oil has gone through various processes that strip away much of its nutritional value. Many chemicals are also used during the processing method. This oil is fine for cooking as many of the unwanted chemicals will also be burned away during the heating process.

Coconut Oil

Coconut oil is considered a healthy oil since it's derived from coconuts. However, most commercial coconut oil you find on the shelf at your local supermarket has gone through a high-processing system. On top of this, coconut oil is high in saturated fats, which aren't as beneficial as unsaturated fats.

This doesn't mean coconut oil is terrible for you. On the contrary, it can help balance bacteria in the gut, improve metabolism, and increase good cholesterol slightly. Coconut oil is better for you than margarine or lard, but it's best to minimize its use. Numerous studies show that boosting good cholesterol levels increases bad cholesterol even more. If you're going to use coconut oil, choose cold-pressed, unrefined, virgin, or extra-virgin oil. This type will not have been processed using heat while maintaining its nutritional value.

Canola Oil

Canola oil is produced from rapeseed. It's higher in monounsaturated fats and can add extra omega-6 and omega-3s to your diet. Many use this for cooking because it has a high heat point and mild flavor.

Vegetable Oil

Vegetables are one of the most commonly used oils for cooking. It's a mix of oils extracted from various plants. These oils don't have much flavor, which is why they're typically used for frying foods. They're higher in polyunsaturated fats and saturated fats.

Butter

Butter should not be confused with margarine. Though both look the same on supermarket shelves, they're vastly different. Butter can add vitamins A, E, and K to your diet, but it's high in saturated fats.

Essential Oils

While we focused on many cooking oils, it's worth discussing other oils that you probably use on your hair and skin or in other beauty and self-care products.

Essential oils are popular for aromatherapy and gain attention as they can be easily added to do-it-yourself lotion and creams. Like cooking oils, not all essential oils are the same. Pure extracts are carefully removed from plants through evaporation or distillation. These pure extracts have many benefits, from improving sleep and mood to reducing wrinkles and toning the skin. You can create hundreds of different smells and combinations for your perfect beauty blend.

You don't need to spend a fortune on magical creams to improve your hair or skin as you age. Using essential oils can help your skin look younger and your hair be more vibrant at any age. Some of the most beneficial oils for hair and skin health include:

- **Lavender oil:** Widely known for its calming effects and the ability to reduce stress, soothes angry and bruised skin and ease headaches.

- **Peppermint oil:** Can relax the nerves, cure skin disorders, and is excellent for hot flashes and digestion.

- **Tea tree oil:** Can be used as a natural deodorant, hand sanitizer, and it soothes skin inflammation as its anti-viral and anti-fungal.

- **Rosehip oil:** Has anti-inflammatory properties, can increase collagen, helps fight free radicals, and regenerates and heals skin.

Industrials Oils

You may have these types of oils in your kitchen. Often sold as vegetable oils and touted to be heart health, this is deceiving. Vegetable oils are highly processed and high in Omega 6 fatty acids. Many oils can fall into the industry oil category, such as:

- Corn

- Sesame

- Canola

- Sunflower

- Grapeseed

Industrial seed oils undergo various alterations to make them "safe" for human consumption. First, soy, corn, cotton, rapeseed, or safflower seeds are gathered. The seeds then must be heated to extremely high temperatures. When exposed to these high temperatures, the unsaturated fatty acids oxidize, creating harmful byproducts.

After the heat process, the seeds are treated with a petroleum-based solvent to help increase the amount of oil extracted from the seeds. Once the oil is extracted, the seeds are treated with chemicals to deodorize them, as most oils have an unpleasant smell. This deodorizing process creates trans fats. Next, the oil is mixed with various chemicals to make it look more appealing.

When the process is finished, the natural oils have gone through a long process that has added harmful chemicals, byproducts, and chemical residue.

The History of Seed Oils

Oils, like cottonseed oils, were used primarily as fuel but not for the body. They were used as fuel in lamps. In the late 1800s in the United States, cottonseed oils were plentiful. William Proctor and James Gamble first decided to use excess cottonseed oils for other means, like making soap. Before this, soap was made from rendered pork fat. Proctor and Gamble experimented with using the oil for soapmaking, discovering that it could be chemically altered through hydrogenation. Hydrogenation is a process that transforms cottonseed oil into a lard-like substance, and products like Crisco were soon born.

As cottonseed oil had little use, what was once considered toxic waste soon transformed the American diet. Crisco was first marketed in the early 1900s, followed by soybean oils in the 1930s, quickly becoming the most popular oil in kitchens around the country. Canola and corn oils were low-cost oils that began populating home kitchens from the 1950s on. After the 1950s, what was once marketed as industrial seed oils became better known as vegetable oils, but this is not where the story ends.

Remember how these seeds were initially classified as "toxic waste?" But today, many of these oils are labeled as "heart healthy." And no, scientists didn't perform many tests that determined they were packed with nutrients and had magical antioxidant powers.

In the 1940s, scientific research was done, possibly because of the $1.5 million donation from Proctor and Gamble. Around the same time, Ancel Keys, a prolific physiologist, conducted his own research that suggested animal fats rich in dietary saturated fats had a negative impact on cholesterol and labeled them as unhealthy. Keys went on to recommend the consumption of polyunsaturated fats, which he concluded reduced cholesterol. Keys' statements aligned with Proctor and Gamble's motives: to get more people to consume more seed oils instead of animal fats. They began running ads stating margin and other seed oils were "heart healthy."

What fueled this fire of getting people to consume more industrial oils was that the National Cholesterol Education Program and the National Institutes of Health had agreed that animal fats were bad for health. They, too, began suggesting a switch to vegetable oils. For decades, people believed that consuming more vegetable seed oils was better than consuming natural oils like butter.

It wasn't until 2014 that analysis of the research conducted in previous years indicated that replacing saturated fat with vegetable oils had no health benefits. However, additional research has since been conducted showing the adverse effect these highly processed vegetable oils have on one's health.

We now know that Keys' original research was heavily flawed. What people latched onto was a hypothesis that was never adequately tested. The companies that could afford to conduct any research were those obtaining donations from Proctor and Gamble, who financially benefited from people consuming industrial oils like Crisco.

Why Industrial Seed Oils Are Bad For Your Health

People bought into the statements that industrial oils were heart-healthy. However, few understand what this means. Heart health refers to the ability of not just the heart to function properly, but the blood vessels' ability to move blood through the body and the fluidity of the blood.

We now know there are many reasons why industrial seed oils are the opposite of healthy. The first is simply that industrial seed oil goes against what our bodies are naturally and biologically designed to process.

Industrial seed oils affect omega-6 and omega-3 fatty acids. They contain significantly more omega-6 and very little, if any, omega-3. Omega-6 raises pro-inflammatory markers, whereas omega-3s raise anti-inflammatory markers. When we consume more omega-6 fatty acids, we can develop chronic inflammation, leading to various chronic health problems.

Another primary concern with industrial seed oils is that when these oils are exposed to heat, trans fats and lipid peroxides are created. Trans fats, as we know, are detrimental to our health. Lipid peroxides are toxic byproducts. They damage your DNA, protein molecules, and membrane lipids. When they accumulate in the body, they contribute to developing chronic disease and triggering the aging process.

These oils go through repeated heat treatments, making them full of toxic byproducts before you use them. In addition, frequent heating depletes their nutrient value, which is already quite low as the oils are retrieved from genetically modified plants. As the natural nutrients in oils deplete, there is an increase in free radicals. These free radicals contribute to the formation of oxidative stress, which causes a wide range of health issues, like high blood pressure, heart disease, and liver damage.

Industrial seed oils also contain additives that are harmful to your health. Synthetic antioxidants, like BHA, BHT, and TBHQ, are added to stop oxidation and prolong the oil's shelf life. Unfortunately, these additives disrupt the endocrine system and hinder the immune system. TBHQ, specifically, can increase the risk of developing food allergies, and it triggers the release of antibodies.

What Oils and Fats Do You Need?

Not all fats from oils are the same, which is why oils are misunderstood. Many lump all oils into the same not-so-good-for-you category. While some should be avoided, others should be included in a balanced diet.

Oils are high in calories, but these calories fuel the body. Therefore, it's recommended that fat should account for 20% to 30% of your daily calorie intake. The quality of fat you consume is more important than the quantity in most cases. Consuming a diet high in saturated fats, even if you stick to the dietary recommendation, is going to result in poor health. However, getting your recommended fat intake from unsaturated fats will help keep you in optimal health.

Unsaturated Fats

Most unsaturated fats are obtained from plant sources, like olives, nuts, and seeds, but some are also obtained from fish. These oils are often in liquid form, making them move easily through the body and causing build-up in your arteries. There are two primary types of unsaturated fat: monounsaturated and polyunsaturated.

Monounsaturated Fats

Extra-virgin olive oil is the best source of monounsaturated fats. These fats can help improve cholesterol levels.

Polyunsaturated Fats

Pure vegetable oils are the best sources of polyunsaturated fats. Polyunsaturated fats are either omega-3 fatty acids or omega-6 fatty acids. We need these fatty acids for proper bodily function, but you want to focus on consuming higher amounts of omega-3 fatty acids as opposed to omega-6 fatty acids. Omega-3 fatty acids are essential for optimal brain health. Omega-6 fatty acids help reduce bad cholesterol, but when consumed in high quantities, they will also lower good cholesterol levels.

Polyunsaturated fats are also essential for hormone production, muscle movement, and cognitive function.

Saturated Fats

It is recommended that you consume less than 10% of your daily calories from saturated fats—or no more than 13 grams. Consuming high amounts of saturated fats can increase the risk of heart disease as it's linked to harmful cholesterol levels. Organic virgin coconut oil has the highest levels of saturated fats. Saturated fats come in solid form and are more likely to clog arteries.

Trans Fats

Trans fats are considered harmful to the body and are some of the worst fats for you. Many food companies have been banned from using them in their products, but this doesn't stop them from sneaking them in. Trans fats are created when hydrogen is added to vegetable oil, resulting in an oil with a longer shelf life. Many food companies use partially hydrogenated oil in their foods because it also prolongs pre-packed items' shelf life.

You can check if an item has trans fats by reading the food label. If you see any form of partially hydrogenated oil listed on the ingredients label, the food contains some amount of trans fat. The United States Federal Drug Administration allows companies to list 0 under the trans-fat component of the nutrient labels if there are less than 0.5 grams of trans fat in the food. While this may seem like an insignificant amount, it quickly adds up when you consume multiple items with less than 0.5 grams of trans fat per serving.

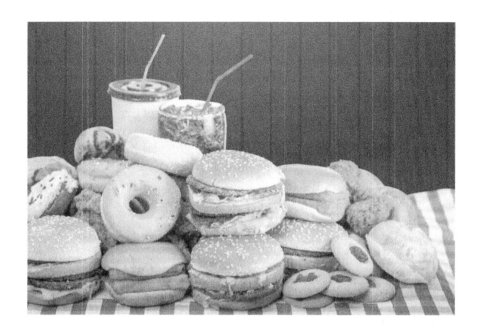

Fat Versus Cholesterol

Fat and cholesterol are types of lipids that are insoluble in water. While fat and cholesterol are closely tied to one another, they perform specific key functions throughout the body, and only a handful of these are similar. For instance, fat is used as an energy source in the body. Cholesterol is not.

Cholesterol is a chemical produced by the liver. Nearly 80% of the cholesterol in your body comes from the liver, and the other 20% is consumed through the foods you eat. High saturated fats increase cholesterol levels. Cholesterol plays many roles in the body. It's present in every cell of our body and is essential for the health of cell membranes. Cholesterol is also needed to create vitamin D and hormones in the body that keep your bones, teeth, and muscles healthy. It also plays a role in the digestive tract.

LDL and HDL Cholesterol

Low-density lipoprotein (LDL) cholesterol is considered bad cholesterol. LDL cholesterol's main job is to carry cholesterol to the cells. LDL contains high amounts of cholesterol so it can disrupt enough of all the cells in the body. However, when there are high LDL cholesterol levels, your arteries can become clogged because too much cholesterol is distributed to the cells. The body needs a small amount of LDL cholesterol in the blood, but we often have significantly more than our body needs.

High-density lipoprotein (HDL) cholesterol is known as good cholesterol. Its primary job is to carry excess cholesterol away from the cells in your body and back to the liver. HDL cholesterol contains more protein, making it denser. Once the cholesterol returns to the liver, it's broken down and expelled or released back into the blood to help aid in digestion.

Low-Fat Versus Full-Fat

How often have you gone into the store and bought low-fat foods because you thought they're better for you? What about that light yogurt you purchased? But you probably didn't ask yourself what was added to replace the fat in that product.

Low-fat foods often have higher quantities of carbohydrates, not the complex kind that slowly breaks down in your body. So when you see low-fat, you can translate this to high carb. High-carb foods will increase triglycerides, which, in simple terms, are the fat that builds up in your body. So if you've been eating low-fat foods to help lose weight, you're actually sabotaging your efforts with low-fat foods.

Additionally, low-fat foods often lack fiber and protein. These two components are what help suppress hunger and keep you feeling full for longer periods. So not only are you increasing your chance to gain weight by eating low-fat, but you'll also often feel the need to eat more, which is counterproductive to any weight loss plan.

Full-fat foods can be better for you, but you must be mindful of where this fat comes from. Avocados, nuts, seeds, olive oil, and fatty fish are great full-fat food sources. Eating these foods can be beneficial to the heart and overall health. Also, most full-fat foods contain higher amounts of protein and fiber. Consuming full-fat products takes your body longer to digest them, which keeps you feeling full for longer.

When making a choice between low-fat or full-fat, it's often better to go with full-fat. But sometimes you might want to consider another alternative. For instance, instead of going with low-fat yogurt, choose plain Greek yogurt, which isn't loaded with sugar and contains more protein. Another example is milk. Many choose skim or low-fat milk, but these aren't much better than regular full-fat options. Even plant-based milk doesn't provide much more protein, though it will have fewer calories and fat. Using kefir milk is the best alternative as it also contains beneficial probiotics, which you'll learn are essential for gut health!

In the next chapter, we'll combine everything you've just learned about what you eat, including oils and fats, to further your health. You will learn how to combat one of the most common causes for serious health conditions: *inflammation*.

Chapter 3:

Boost Your Immune System by

Fighting Inflammation

What is the one thing most individuals with Alzheimer's, diabetes, and heart disease have in common?

Chronic inflammation.

Inflammation doesn't get enough focus when it comes to improving overall health. However, it's one of the most common conditions that cause serious mental and physical health conditions. Fighting inflammation begins by improving your gut health, which is done through diet.

Bringing Awareness to Inflammation

We often don't think about how that sore wrist, aching back, or tight knees can be more serious than just overuse. These obvious indicators of inflammation are just one way the body fights off infection and heals from an injury. When the immune system identifies a cut, bacteria, or virus in the body, it releases chemicals that cause more blood to flow to the infected area to begin the healing process. You feel the immune response throughout your body. A cut may burn or feel hot, your joints may feel swollen, or you have frequent muscle aches. They are signs that the immune system is responding to an injury in the body. When a foreign item is found in the body, the immune system sends out a message to identify unwanted invaders in the body and how to remove them.

The driving force of an immune response is cytokines. These messages are sent between immune cells to rid the body of the foreign invader effectively. However, communication in the immune system can be disrupted or go astray, resulting in the system triggering an immune response when one isn't needed. This causes inflammation to occur where there's no threat. When our body is frequently in an inflammatory response, it can cause chaos in other systems. Suffering from acute or chronic inflammation signals that your immune system is working in overdrive.

Acute Versus Chronic Inflammation

Acute inflammation is often managed with over-the-counter medication, like ibuprofen or acetaminophen. It's normal to experience acute inflammation from time to time, but it becomes a major concern when this becomes persistent and almost daily. Low-grade inflammation of this sort, when experienced more frequently, is considered chronic inflammation. Many factors can contribute to chronic inflammation, such as smoking, overweight, stress, and poor diet. If not properly managed, this inflammation can cause more severe conditions like diabetes, cancer, arthritis, and even heart disease.

Unfortunately, acute, chronic inflammation isn't always noticeable. You might not be aware for months or even years that you're experiencing it. Inflammation can also show itself in other ways, not just from aches and pains. Certain skin conditions, like psoriasis and eczema, can result from inflammation. Cognitive impairments can also result from high inflammatory markers in the body. While inflammation can impact various areas of the body, communication around whether to launch an inflammatory response begins in one general area. To better understand how inflammation affects your body, we need to understand why or where the signals come from in the first place.

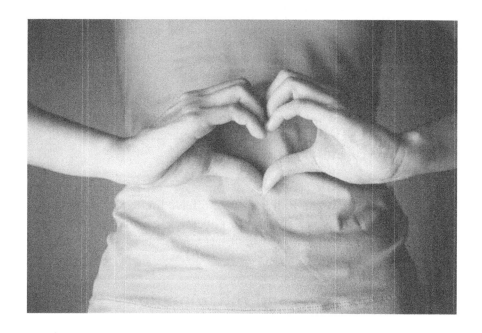

Gut Health and Inflammation

The immune systems trigger inflammation. A large portion of the immune system is located in the digestive tract. The digestive tract is often misunderstood simply because many people only associate it with the stomach and intestine, but it runs almost the entire body length starting at the mouth. Because it's a long-running system, it comes in direct and indirect contact with many of our primary organs and other major processes in the body. The digestive tract has many roles, so it's vital to focus on maintaining a healthy gut.

A healthy gut is more specific to the stomach's microbiome and the type of bacteria that lives there. The digestive tract is home to billions of bacteria. This bacteria is responsible for extracting essential nutrients from the foods you consume. It also aids in hormone production so the body can adequately absorb the nutrients released. The gut needs a diverse growth of different bacteria. Some are considered beneficial, and others are deemed bad. Both types of bacteria are essential for a healthy gut, but microbiome health issues arise when bad bacteria are the majority of the gut.

When it comes to inflammation, the gut has a significant influence. When there's an overgrowth of certain bacteria, inflammatory molecules are released. They trigger inflammation in various parts of the body, causing disruption. The gut bacteria have the power to activate or prevent inflammation.

Maintaining a robust gut microbiome is crucial for reducing inflammation in the body. Individuals who have limited variation in gut bacteria are more likely to suffer from allergies, eczema, diabetes, and obesity.

Diet, Gut Bacteria, and Inflammation

While there's still a lot to learn about the gut microbiome's intricacies, we know that the type of bacteria impacts how the body operates. Bacteria are responsible for processing the foods we eat and transforming them into different compounds that can be used and are essential for the body. We know that the foods we consume directly impact what types of bacteria will flourish in the gut and which will be weeded out. You'll learn about the direct connection between the type of bacteria that thrives in the digestive tract, the food you eat, and inflammation.

Friendly or "Good" Bacteria

Good bacteria are classified as those that produce short-chain fatty acids. These acids help control the inflammation response when the gut bacteria release these acids; they aid in protecting the lining of the gut.

Healthy bacteria rely on soluble and insoluble fiber. Eating a plant-based diet and consuming more fermented foods can promote the growth of good anti-inflammatory bacteria.

Unfriendly or "Bad Bacteria

Bad bacteria produce many harmful chemicals, which include pro-inflammatory chemicals. In addition, when the digestive tract has an abundance of bad bacteria, other bacteria, which would otherwise be harmless, begin to cause additional health problems because of a weakened immune system.

Bad bacteria flourish when an abundance of simple sugars, simple carbohydrates, and other ingredients in processed foods are consumed. This bacteria will also damage and feed on the mucus of the intestinal walls, which can cause toxins to be released into the bloodstream.

Gut-Healthy Foods

To maintain a healthy gut, you want to focus on consuming foods that will feed and support the growth of the more beneficial bacteria. Eating plenty of fruits and vegetables can help keep the gut microbiota diverse.

Eating fermented foods, like sauerkraut, yogurt, and kefir, provide a healthy dose of probiotics. Probiotics contain live microorganisms that will take up home in your gut.

Antibiotics kill off a majority of gut bacteria, both good and bad. That's why after taking antibiotics, it's recommended to take a probiotic. Probiotics promote the process of beneficial bacteria regrowth.

Anti-Inflammatory Foods

Since gut bacteria is affected by the foods we eat, we can adjust our diet to consume more anti-inflammatory foods. These foods feed the good bacteria and help minimize the presence of bad bacteria in the gut. An anti-inflammatory diet is not complex to follow and will have profound positive effects on your overall health.

Anti-Inflammatory Diet

An anti-inflammatory diet focuses on consuming foods with key nutrients that combat inflammation. For instance, fruits, vegetables, and organic teas contain high quantities of antioxidants and phytochemicals to help eliminate chemicals that can trigger an inflammatory response. More anti-inflammatory foods to eat more of include:

- Apples

- Blueberries

- Strawberries

- Oranges

- Cherries

- Tomatoes

- Yellow vegetable (squash, bell pepper)

- Spinach

- Kale

- Nuts

- Olive oil

- Fatty fish (salmon, sardines, tuna)

High-fiber diets also help minimize inflammation as they help promote a healthy gut. In addition, fiber is an essential food source for healthy bacteria.

Anti-inflammatory diets discourage consuming inflammation-promoting foods, such as:

- Refined carbohydrates

- Fried foods

- Refined sugars

- Red meats

- Processed meats

- Saturated fats (margarin, lard, shortening)

Mediterranean Diet

The Mediterranean Diet is a prime example of an anti-inflammatory diet. It has been touted as one of the most beneficial diets for overall health. It also emphasizes eating some of the best anti-inflammatory foods, like fruits, vegetables, and fish. The Mediterranean Diet mimics the eating habits of those living around the Mediterranean Sea up until the 1950s. The people living here were once considered the healthiest people in the world. When the habits of these people were looked at, it was clear their diet played an integral role in better health.

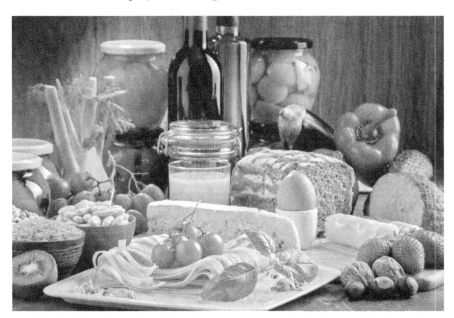

The Mediterranean Diet has five primary foods staples:

- Seasonal fruits and vegetables

- Fish

- Whole grains

- Olive oil

- Nuts and seeds

While red meats are consumed in this diet, they are incorporated sparingly.

These foods help promote a diverse and rich microbiome with plenty of good bacteria and anti-inflammatory bacteria flourishing. Aside from the anti-inflammatory benefits, you should know the Mediterranean Diet has been shown to combat cardiovascular disease, diabetes, and metabolic syndrome.

The benefits of an anti-inflammatory diet are accelerated when combined with intermittent fasting. In the next chapter, you'll learn how intermittent fasting can improve your overall health after 50.

Chapter 4:

How Can You Benefit From

Intermittent Fasting?

Intermittent fasting is popular because of its effectiveness in helping you lose weight. But, how much weight can you lose by intermittent fasting?

Several studies have shown that, on average, you can lose between 3% to 7% of your body weight in just eight weeks through intermittent fasting (Alexis, 2022).

Weight loss isn't the only reason you want to consider sticking to a fasting plan. There has been more and more evidence and research showing that fasting can improve many functions of the body. However, like any appealing diet plan, there is a wrong and a right way to have the most success with intermittent fasting.

What Is Intermittent Fasting?

Intermittent fasting (IF) is an eating plan that utilizes an eating and fasting window. It doesn't restrict the foods you eat. Instead, it limits the time you have throughout the day to eat. You can eat whatever you want, but only in a specific time frame, referred to as "the eating window." While most diet plans you've been on probably set up guidelines and restrictions around **what** you eat, intermittent fasting establishes **when** you eat.

There are different eating windows you can try. There is no one-size-fits-all when it comes to fasting. Some people excel with an eight-hour eating window; others find it harder to stick to this timeframe but do well with a 10- or 12-hour window.

Intermittent fasting works by assisting your body to burn fat instead of relying on a constant stream of fuel. It helps rewire your body for how it was programmed to consume foods, not for hours on end but for specific periods. Consider back to our ancestors who had to hunt and gather food, or even 50 years ago when there weren't as many convenience foods. We could last hours, even days, without eating and not feel incredibly hungry. Now, because we're so used to having meals ready at the push of a button or in a short amount of time, going hours without eating causes us stress and some anxiety.

You can eat just one meal a day (OMAD), three large meals a day, or smaller meals with a snack or two in between. So, it's not much different than how most people plan out their meals already.

The difference is that you consume all your food within the eating window, and that's it. No more middle-of-the-night snacking that can cause stress and anxiety.

When you limit the time, you give yourself to eat, your body naturally switches from using up all the sugar or other fuel you consume during the day and instead begins to burn stored fat. So, by shortening the window when you consume calories to fuel your body in, you trigger the natural fat-burning process.

Although there are no strict guidelines for what you can eat during the eating window, eating a variety of nutritious foods will benefit you the most. Conversely, eating highly processed foods or foods lacking nutrients will make it harder to stick with a fasting period.

During your fasting window, consuming items with zero calories is essential. For example, you can drink water, coffee, or tea, as long as the coffee and tea have no sugar, cream, milk, or other flavoring added to them.

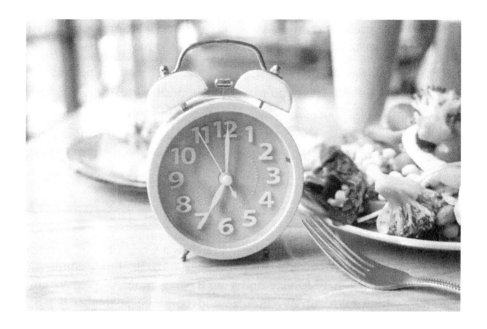

Types of Intermittent Fasting

Intermittent fasting allows you to choose from a time-based eating window or schedule weekly eating windows. Below you'll find an explanation of some of the most common IF plans to consider.

Time-Restricted

Time-restricted fasts establish a strict number of hours you fast and a strict number of hours you eat. Many people already follow a restricted eating schedule as they fast while sleeping. However, this period is extended when you begin intermittent fasting. This is a great option for those interested in getting started with intermittent fasting.

The most common time-restricted fasting approaches are:

- 16/8, where you fast for 16 hours and have an eating window of eight hours. Begin by picking an eight-hour eating window; some popular times are 9 a.m.-5 p.m., noon-8 p.m., or 2-10 p.m.

Many prefer the noon-10 p.m. window, as skipping breakfast and consuming two well-balanced meals is more manageable.

- 14/10, where you fast for 14 hours and have an eating window of 10 hours. This type may be beneficial for early risers. You can begin your eating window at 7 a.m. and finish your last meal at 5 p.m. The eating window closes, and you continue the fast until 7 a.m. the next day.

Twice-a-Week Method

This fasting plan lets you eat regularly five days a week and fast for two days. Your fasting days should not be back-to-back. For example, if you fast from 9 p.m. Monday and your fasting time is up at 9 p.m. Tuesday, you would skip Wednesday and continue fasting at 9 p.m. Wednesday for 24 hours.

An alternative to this approach is the 5:2 approach. This is similar to the twice-a-week method described above, but on your "fasting days," you restrict your calorie intake to no more than 500 calories a day.

Alternate Day Fasting

Alternate fasting combines the twice-a-week and 5:2 methods. Every other day, you restrict your calorie intake to 500 to 600 calories and eat as you usually would every other day.

24-Hour Fast or Eat. Stop. Eat Method

Similar to alternate day fasting, you eat regularly one day and fast the next. You continue with this plan for the whole week. You can also opt just to do one 24-hour fast a week.

What matters most is that you keep your fasting time consistent. You can lengthen or shorten the eating window, but your fasting time should remain the same. So if you choose a 16/8 fast (fast for 16 hours, eat for eight), you don't have to start your eating window at the same time you did the day before. Sometimes you'll need to adjust the eating window.

For instance, if you know you're going to need to be up earlier the next day and you typically have your first meal at 9 a.m., you can bump up your first meal to 7 a.m., but you would need to move up your last meal from the day before to ensure that you still fast for the total 16 hours. If your regular fasting times are 9 a.m.-5 p.m., when you begin eating at 7 a.m., your last meal would be at 3 p.m., maintaining the 16-hour fast.

Risks

I always recommend speaking to your primary care physician before trying intermittent fasting. While there are many benefits to this eating approach, a few individuals want to get the OK from the doctor before committing. These include:

- Anyone under the age of 18. If you want to get your kids on board with intermittent fasting, this probably isn't the best idea. Young children and teens need more calories and nutrition to support their still-developing bodies.

- Those with diabetes or issues with blood sugar need to understand how to properly manage their glucose levels before trying intermittent fasting.

- If you have a history of eating disorders, such as bulimia, anorexia, or binge eating, you should speak to a professional first. Adhering to an IF schedule can trigger obsessiveness around how much and what you eat.

Even if your doctor says intermittent fasting is appropriate for you, there are other signs to be aware of. If you experience any of the following for a prolonged period, you want to reach out to your doctor:

- Higher levels of anxiety

- Nausea

- Lightheadedness

- Sleeplessness

- Moodiness

- Increase in weight

Any adverse changes after you start the IF approach should be reported to your doctor. These often overlooked symptoms can be an indication of more severe problems.

Benefits of Intermittent Fasting

Intermittent fasting offers a wide range of benefits. While many begin fasting to help lose weight and curb cravings, they can also benefit from the various ways it can help improve overall health.

Balances Hormone Functions

When you begin to fast, your body will undergo many changes in the way it functions. This includes:

- Insulin levels drop as your body begins to use stored fat for fuel.

- The level of human growth hormone (HGH) increases as it's needed to maintain the fat-burning process.

- Cellular waste is eliminated more rapidly, which initiates cellular repair.

Helps Burn Visceral Fat

Visceral fat is harmful because it's stored around the major organs, mainly located deep in the abdomen. Excess visceral fat has been connected with various health problems like heart disease and high cholesterol. When you're fasting, you'll consume fewer calories, triggering the body to burn this excess fat for fuel.

Reduces Risk for Type 2 Diabetes

One of the significant factors that contribute to diabetes is insulin resistance. This occurs when the body can't use the insulin produced by the pancreas to properly absorb the glucose in the body. As a result, the excess glucose that can't be used is stored as fat. When your body consistently has higher insulin levels, you're at a greater risk of developing diabetes.

Helps Remove Free Radicals

Free radicals are unstable and foreign molecules in the body. These molecules have harmful interactions with cells and other healthy normal molecules in the body that can cause damage, oxidative stress, and inflammation. Oxidative stress speeds up the aging process and can play a role in developing chronic disease. Intermittent fasting can help remove and eliminate excess free radicals throughout the body.

Heart Health Benefits

Intermittent fasting can help improve many of the body functions that keep the heart healthy, such as:

- Regulating blood sugar levels

- Improving blood pressure

- Lowering triglyceride levels

- Reducing inflammatory markers

- Lowering bad cholesterol levels

Cellular Waste Removal

Fasting can help trigger autophagy, which removes cellular waste. When the autophagy process increases, you can protect cognitive function and prevent various other harmful health conditions. More information is provided in the next section.

Cancer Prevention

While research needs continuous studying in these areas, there is a positive correlation between fasting and changes in metabolism. The metabolic changes could potentially control the growth of cells that have abnormalities. Additionally, those who adhere to a fasting diet often experience fewer side effects due to chemotherapy.

Improves Brain Health

Many of the benefits previously mentioned also aid in better brain health. Reducing oxidative stress and inflammation can help improve brain function, for instance. Fasting can also increase the levels of brain-derived neurotrophic factors (BDNF). BDNF is a hormone that helps improve mood, reducing the risk of depression. Fasting can also help repair damage caused by stroke and promote new brain cell growth.

Protects Against Alzheimer's

Alzheimer's disease is a devastating neurodegenerative condition without a cure. However, fasting has been shown to improve Alzheimer's symptoms and may help prevent or slow down the onset of this condition.

Extended Life Expectancy

Many favorable studies indicate fasting can prolong one's lifespan. Seeing how fasting can improve key health areas, like the heart and brain, it's clear that this can add more years to your life.

Autophagy and Fasting

Autophagy is another benefit of intermittent fasting. Autophagy translates to self-eating; while it may sound grotesque, it's a naturally occurring process our bodies undergo. During autophagy, the body uses damaged or unnecessary cells to clean and rejuvenate cell growth. Simply put, autophagy is a process that removes cellular waste. This is done so we can maintain a natural state of homeostasis. Homeostasis is when the systems and cells in our body work in harmony.

There are a few key benefits of autophagy. First, when stressed, our cells don't retrieve adequate oxygen and other nutrients. If our body is in autophagy, these stressed cells are supplied with the necessary energy they need from other sources—damaged cells. This provides help to maintain these deprived, yet healthy cells' cellular structure and ultimately keeps them alive. Additionally, autophagy helps support the immune system by clearing away toxins and other harmful intruders.

Increased autophagy can help protect and/or prevent severe health conditions. As we discussed earlier, autophagy helps remove free radicals and can improve cognitive function. Fasting helps trigger autophagy because you eliminate energy sources your cells can use. Our cells often rely on readily available energy, which is dispersed when insulin levels increase due to the intake of carbohydrates. When we cut off these carbohydrates, the body must turn to other energy sources, such as broken-down old damaged cells, for fuel.

The body must experience at least a 14-hour fast for fasting to impact autophagy significantly. Short-term fasting of 24 hours has an even more beneficial impact. However, if you have never tried fasting before, starting with a 24-hour fast or an extended fast—say, for five days—might be far-reaching. Your best option is to stick with a consistent 16-hour fast with an eight-hour eating window. You'll still experience the benefits of autophagy but have a much easier time adhering to a fasting window long enough for the body to work its internal magic.

Fasting for Women Over 50

Women over 50 go through various changes, and as someone approaching 50 or already over 50, you understand that there are more struggles around maintaining an ideal weight. This struggle with your weight is due to the changes in your hormones. While completely natural, it can be frustrating when you feel as though there's nothing you can do to help prevent weight gain and other negative impacts on your body.

Those who are of perimenopause and menopause age know that their estrogen levels begin to drop significantly. With this dip in estrogen, other hormone levels start to change. Cortisol, thyroid, serotonin, and progesterone are all influenced by menopause.

In addition to the many hormonal changes the body goes through, it also shifts how we store fat. Women will find they gain fat around the midsection, hips, and thighs. You might also find losing or maintaining weight harder as you get closer to menopause due to a loss in muscle mass. Losing muscle mass causes the metabolism to slow, so you won't use as many calories as you typically would. Instead, we store excess calories as fat.

It is also common for women to exercise less as they get older. This combination of hormonal changes, distribution of fat, loss of muscle mass, and less physical activity makes it incredibly challenging to lose weight and keep it off.

Intermittent fasting can help counter many issues that cause menopausal women to gain weight. By restricting your eating window, you can reduce the number of calories you consume. Fewer calories mean you won't store excess fat. This also means the body will need to turn to other fuel sources, like your stored fat, to get the energy it needs.

A case study published in *Nutrition, Metabolism, and Cardiovascular Disease* (NMCD) highlights IF benefits for pre-and postmenopausal women.

During a 12-week study, women followed an alternate-day fasting schedule. The study found that premenopausal women lost an average of 4-½ pounds. At the same time, postmenopausal women lost an average of 6-½ pounds. They also notice a more significant decrease in LDL cholesterol in premenopausal women (Lin, et al., 2021).

While this study shows that intermittent fasting can be an efficient way to lose weight, there are other factors you need to understand if you want to have this kind of success.

Unfortunately, your body goes into famine or starvation mode when there is a prolonged period without food. If the body is consistently in starvation mode, it begins to preserve energy, resulting in more fat storage. The body will also produce more ghrelin and leptin, the hunger hormones that cause you to feel more intense hunger episodes. The body will also slow down specific systems or functions, primarily those in the reproductive system.

This doesn't mean you can't have success with intermittent fasting. You just need to know how to properly use this plan to ensure weight loss and a balance of hormones.

Tips for Successful Intermittent Fasting

What you eat during your feeding window will determine how many calories you consume. Fasting can make it easier to consume fewer calories during the day, which makes weight loss possible. However, consuming as many, if not more, calories during your feeding window is possible if you aren't sticking to nutritious foods. When you begin intermittent fasting, stick with the following foods to ensure a healthy journey:

- High-fiber foods and lean proteins, such as whole grains, vegetables, poultry, and fish, will help you feel fuller for longer, so you'll consume fewer calories during your eating window.

- Healthy fats, such as extra virgin olive oil, avocados, and coconut oil, can help keep your brain sharp and focused.

- Colorful fruits and vegetables, such as blueberries, kale, and bell peppers, that contain high amounts of polyphenols will help combat inflammation.

Each of these can keep your caloric intake down, making it easier to lose weight while also experiencing the other benefits of a nutritious diet. When your fasting window is over, it's recommended your first meal be lean protein and fiber-rich carbohydrates, such as baked chicken breast and quinoa. This type of eating allows you to feel—and stay—full for many hours quickly.

You can consume zero-calorie drinks, such as water, tea, or black coffee, during your fasting window. You can't eat any food during your fasting window. All foods contain calories, which will break your fast, negating the progress you've made. If you struggle to get through those last few hours of your fasting window, drinking hot tea or coffee can help you push through. Just be sure not to add any milk, cream, or sugar. The warmth of the coffee or tea can give the impression that your belly is full and can help combat hunger.

It's important not to break your fast. This is the period in which your body will begin to use up the stored energy it has, and this is how you can drop the fat.

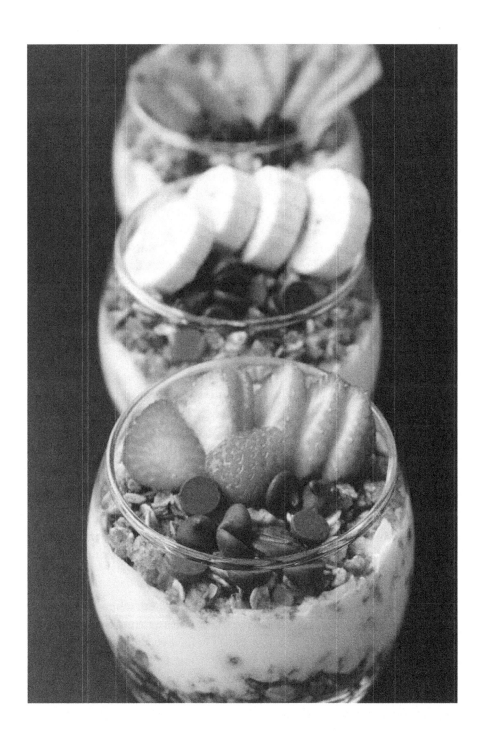

Finding the Right IF Schedule for You

Intermittent fasting should be an easy-to-follow eating habit. You shouldn't ever feel uncomfortable or deprived during your fasting periods. While some women find fasting for 16 or even 20 hours easy, others find it more depleting. The best fasting plan for you is one you can consistently stick to without feeling deprived. It may take a few weeks to get to this point on your fasting plan, but allow yourself to commit to one method for a few weeks before determining it's working for you. You won't see a miraculous shift in your weight, energy, or health overnight. But, after a few weeks, you'll notice the changes. There are plenty of ways you can get through the first few weeks with more ease and enjoyment.

Choosing the Right IF Plan for You

There are some signs you'll notice whether you're on the right IF plan. Three key factors to consider are ease, schedule, and overall health goals.

When considering the ease of fasting, you want to focus on how comfortable you feel while you're fasting. You should expect some hunger during your fasting time, but you shouldn't feel so hungry that you eat uncontrollably during your eating window. Additionally, other areas of your health should improve, not feel worse. Experiencing new or worsening symptoms, such as trouble sleeping or irritability, can indicate that you need to shorten your fasting time.

The second consideration, time, is often neglected when choosing a fasting time. Fasting should give you more freedom, but for intermittent fasting to work correctly, you need to find the right schedule that works for you. You don't want to commit to a fasting schedule that will disrupt important times in your life. For instance, if eating dinner together as a family is quality time, then thinking that an alternate-day fasting schedule will work will set you up for disappointment. Instead, consider an alternative schedule if you feel like fasting is taking away valuable time.

Know what your goals are for choosing a fasting schedule. Many try intermittent fasting to lose weight, improve overall health, or take control of their eating habits. A clear goal for starting a fasting program can help you decide the best schedule. Those trying to lose weight will benefit more from longer fasting windows to increase the body's natural process for burning fat and to decrease the total number of calories you consume during the eating window. However, longer fasting times may diminish muscle mass which can be counterproductive if you want to burn more calories while working out.

It's important to keep this in mind: Fasting for longer periods—24 hours or longer—isn't going to reap more benefits. With longer fasting times, there comes the risk of having a harder time maintaining muscle mass. For those over 50, this is already a common concern, even when not fasting.

Tips to Maintain Intermittent Fasting

If you have tried intermittent fasting or found it hard to jump right into a long fasting window, you should work up to a longer fasting time. Begin by sticking to a week where you fast for 12 hours a day. Stop eating two hours before bed, sleep eight hours and eat two hours after you wake up. That's a 12-hour fast. The following week, add an extra hour to your fast. Continue adding an extra hour to your fasting window until you reach a comfortable period. For some, it may be 14 hours; for others, it may be 18. If you feel uncomfortable at any point, drop back down to the most recent fasting time before that week. For instance, if your current week is a 15-hour fasting window, but you're experiencing adverse effects, go back to a 14-hour fasting time.

Remember, the goal isn't to go as long as possible without eating. Instead, it is to maintain a sustainable fasting window you can stick with long-term.

Be mindful of what you eat. Intermittent fasting will not provide as many benefits if you constantly consume high-calorie, low-nutrient foods. Eating a well-balanced, nutrient-rich diet will allow you to accomplish your health goals.

To help maintain muscle, you should focus on consuming plenty of lean proteins and add strength training to your weekly schedule. These two will ensure your muscles are properly cared for and kept in optimal shape.

When Intermittent Fasting Isn't Right for You

If you're adamant about sticking to an IF method, you should be aware of some signs that it may not be the right fit for you. For example, if you feel or have the following symptoms at any point, you want to consider taking a different approach to fasting.

- Trouble sleeping.

- Negative mood during your fasting window.

- Unable to exercise at the same level as before you started intermittent fasting.

- You feel physically weak.

- You're more tired than usual.

- You're experiencing higher levels of stress since you began fasting.

- You develop an odd resentment towards others when they eat in front of you when you're fasting.

Remember, it's OK if intermittent fasting doesn't work for you. For some, it works wonders, but for others, not so much. This doesn't mean you should give up on your quest for optimal health. It just means you need to travel a different path to get there.

One of the things that you can do to help optimize your health is to keep your blood sugar levels in check. We often think that our blood sugars are only affected by sugar, but they are just one factor that can cause our sugar levels to rise above healthy levels.

Chapter 5:

Why You Need to Monitor Glucose

Levels

Many only become concerned with their glucose levels when they hear the word "diabetes." Only when blood sugar levels remain too high do we begin to cut back on the foods that spike these levels. However, neglected glucose levels, whether too high or low, can wreak havoc on your health. As you get older, years of consuming foods high in sugar and carbohydrates make it even harder to keep blood sugar levels in check.

Managing glucose levels isn't something you should put off or not be concerned with simply because you're not at high risk for diabetes. High glucose levels can lead to many unwanted conditions, all of which can be prevented.

What Is Glucose?

Glucose is a monosaccharide (one sugar) carbohydrate. It's the body's primary source of fuel. All carbohydrates and sugars are converted into glucose so the body can properly use them as fuel for our muscles and cells. When there is an excess of glucose, it is stored as fat.

When speaking about glucose in the body, it's also often referred to as blood sugar. The pancreas helps break down the carbohydrates we consume by producing insulin to manage our blood sugar levels. Without insulin, the cells, muscles, and tissues in the body cannot take in glucose.

Why Glucose Should Be Monitored

Glucose levels fluctuate throughout the day. Normal glucose levels fall between 80 to 130 mg/dL after two or more hours between eating or during fasting times. One to two hours after a meal, glucose levels will rise but should remain under 180 mg/dL. When and what you eat will cause levels to increase more. Exercising will also influence your glucose levels. A continuous glucose monitor will assist you in determining whether your blood sugar levels are within a healthy range.

The body can have difficulty processing glucose when the pancreas cannot properly produce insulin. As a result, type 2 diabetes develops, resulting in the need for medication and possibly insulin injections to regulate blood sugar levels and to assist the body in processing glucose.

Insulin resistance, a precursor to diabetes, is another condition where the body can't absorb glucose. With insulin resistance, it's the insulin that the body doesn't recognize. Without insulin, the cells can't use glucose, keeping blood sugar levels high. Since the cells still need fuel but can't use glucose, they trigger the release of ketones. The liver releases ketones, which typically occurs overnight or while fasting because food isn't being consumed. However, when this happens frequently and not just through the evening hours when you're supposed to be sleeping, insulin resistance keeps insulin levels too low. More ketones are triggered, lowering the blood pH to an acidic level.

Over time, ketones can begin to build up in the body. When combined with higher acidity, ketoacidosis can occur. Ketoacidosis can be fatal and requires immediate medical attention.

A fasting blood sugar level of 99 mg/dL or lower is average, 100 to 125 mg/dL indicates you have prediabetes, and 126 mg/dL or higher indicates you have diabetes. Remember that if you have diabetes, your "normal" glucose levels will differ from those not diagnosed with this condition. If you have diabetes, your fasting glucose levels will be around 100 mg/dL and around 140 mg/dL up to two hours after eating.

You may not be concerned about your glucose levels but should be aware of the risk factors that can lead to type 2 diabetes. These include:

- Being diagnosed with prediabetes.

- If you are overweight.

- If you are over the age of 45.

- If you have a family history of diabetes.

- Engage in little physical activity—less than three times a week.

- If you were diagnosed with gestational diabetes or had a baby weighing over nine pounds.

- If you have a history of nonalcoholic fatty liver disease.

Fluctuation in Glucose

Hyperglycemia can occur when glucose levels are consistently above 130 mg/dL, indicating your body isn't producing enough insulin to manage glucose. After a meal, glucose levels shouldn't be higher than 180 mg/dL. Two clear signs that you might be hyperglycemic are frequent urination and excessive thirst.

High glucose levels are always a concern, but low glucose levels can also cause health problems. Glucose levels below 70 mg/dL are a red flag of hypoglycemia. Symptoms of hypoglycemia include:

- Anxiety

- Confusion

- Fatigue

- Sweating

- Tremors

Lower glucose levels can be due to excessive exercise or not eating enough calories throughout the day. Low glucose can be regulated by eating or drinking a little juice. If ignored, hypoglycemia can become fatal.

Other Fluctuation Causes

The foods we eat are the primary factors that cause glucose levels to fluctuate. However, you should be aware of other things that can shift your blood sugar levels.

- If you have a sunburn, it can put extra stress on the body, which can drive up glucose levels.

- If you've consumed coffee in the past 24 hours, your glucose levels may be slightly higher depending on how sensitive you are to caffeine. Even if you drink black coffee, your blood sugar may rise.

- Not eating breakfast can increase your blood glucose levels more than after you eat lunch and dinner.

- Blood sugar levels may rise in the early morning due to a surge of hormones produced once the body wakes up.

- Certain medications, like nasal sprays, can increase blood glucose levels.

- High levels of stress can cause glucose levels to increase.

If glucose levels go unregulated for too long, many complications can occur. Some symptoms you might experience include:

- Numbness in the hands or feet

- Tingling of the hands and feet

- Loss of sight

- Skin infections

- Extreme pain in the joints

- Dehydration

- Coma

As previously discussed, those with diabetes can suffer conditions such as ketoacidosis, hyperglycemia, hypoglycemia, and hyperosmolar syndrome (HHS). HHS occurs when your glucose levels remain alarmingly high for a long time. Severe confusion or cognitive issues, extreme thirst and dehydration, seizures, and organ failure can occur if untreated.

If glucose levels go unchecked, severe health conditions will also arise. Heart disease, stroke, nerve damage, and kidney disease can result from not monitoring glucose levels properly if you have diabetes.

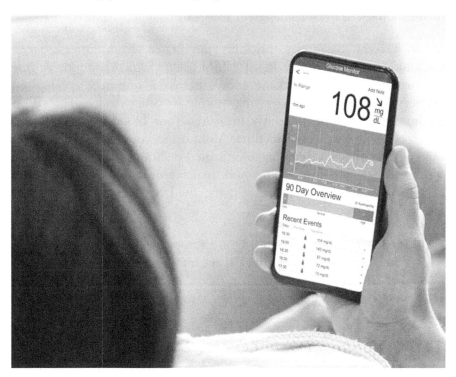

How to Monitor Glucose Levels

When you monitor glucose levels, you can identify what causes your blood sugar levels to fall too far out of range. Tracking your levels and what influences glucose levels can help you learn to avoid things that can cause levels that are too high or low. By detecting irregular glucose levels early, you can prevent the development of more complicated conditions like type 2 diabetes.

Glucose levels are measured using a glucose monitor, and different activities can impact how high or low blood sugar reads. Those with diabetes often need to monitor their blood sugar levels frequently throughout the day. A blood test that requires you to prick your finger and test the blood using a testing strip and a glucose monitor can measure the glucose in the body. This requires taking readings before and after sleeping, eating, exercising, traveling, taking other medications, or a drastic change in your daily schedule.

If you have an aversion to pricking your finger several times a day, a continuous glucose monitor, or CGM, is a painless option. A tiny sensor placed on the back of your arm has a tiny needlepoint that wirelessly sends a signal to a smartphone or other device. The CGM automatically and continuously measures your blood sugar, enabling you to check your levels anytime. Monitoring your blood sugar with this method allows you to make informed decisions on balancing your food, exercise, physical activity, and medication in real time. This type of sensor measures the glucose in the fluid between the cells, called interstitial glucose.

An A1C test conducted from a blood sample will give you an idea of your average glucose levels over three months. Those with diabetes have this test performed once or twice a year. If you're concerned about your risk of developing diabetes, you can request an A1C.

Taking Control of Your Glucose Levels

Managing your glucose levels does not have to be an overwhelming or stressful task. Many find that eating a well-balanced diet and getting a little more exercise is enough to keep their glucose levels in a normal range. Being aware of what you eat can help you take control and avoid serious health concerns.

Being mindful of the carbs you consume is a significant first step to managing glucose levels. The body converts all carbohydrates into glucose, which all cells use for energy. However, not all carbs are processed the same way. Some carbohydrates are rapidly broken down and sent out to the body immediately, while others are slowly broken down and released in a steady stream.

Simple carbs include foods like white bread, pasta, and rice. Soda, pop, sugary drinks, white sugar, and syrups are also simple carbs. Complex carbs include whole grains, fruits, and vegetables. Swapping your simple carbs for complex cards, such as eating whole grain bread instead of white bread, is an easy step you can take to manage glucose levels better.

Sleep and Glucose

As you sleep, your glucose levels fluctuate, rising and falling slightly during different stages of sleep. If your circadian rhythm is regulated, the increases and decreases in blood sugar levels aren't a concern. The circadian rhythm is the body's internal clock that naturally lets you rest, become alert, and is often controlled by light. During sleep, the body goes through several processes to heal, organize memories and new information, and replenish hormones. If our circadian rhythm is out of sync, many essential processes that help us function get out of sync, including regulating our blood sugar levels.

Over the years, sleep has become less and less important in today's busy society. It's become an unfortunate badge of honor to admit that we've only gotten a few hours of sleep every night. With this loss of sleep, there's a greater risk of becoming obese and developing diabetes. Various factors contribute to blood sugar levels imbalanced due to lack of sleep, including:

- Lack of sleep increases cortisol levels, which increases glucose levels.

- Lack of sleep causes a decrease in insulin sensitivity which causes glucose levels to be harder to regulate.

- When sleep impacts cortisol and insulin levels. Cortisol and insulin levels drop a few hours after you sleep and peak a few hours before you wake. If you're sleeping during the day, you're causing levels to drop, which will eventually rise later in the day. This can make getting to sleep harder in the evening.

- Lack of sleep increases inflammation in the body, which affects glucose.

- Oxidative stress increases when we don't get enough sleep, which has a negative impact on glucose levels.

It's important to understand the relationship between sleep and glucose levels is a two-way street. Sleep affects glucose levels, and glucose levels impact sleep. For instance, those with type 2 diabetes have been known to have more troubled sleep patterns when their blood sugar levels are elevated. Individuals with blood sugar levels in the normal range tend to have more quality sleep (Pacheco, 2022).

Properly managing glucose throughout the day and while you sleep is essential. Sleep plays an integral role in a healthy lifestyle, and women over 50 may experience more disturbed sleep as their bodies go through various changes. Intermittent fasting can help keep glucose levels in check as you sleep, which can lead to quality sleep for menopausal women.

Intermittent Fasting for Better Sleep

Intermittent fasting can help regulate your circadian rhythm and bring it into its natural setting. While light is the primary factor that triggers different processes of the circadian rhythm, food is a close second in helping regulate your internal clocks. Intermittent fasting helps you stick to a more scheduled eating plan, leading to a more restful sleep.

Intermittent fasting establishes a more natural sleep cycle. When you're fasting, there's an increase in the production of the human growth hormone (HGH). This hormone is also naturally produced while you sleep, so syncing your fasting time with your sleep cycle results in higher HGH levels. Human growth hormone is beneficial because it helps burn fat, repairs muscles, and heals the body on a cellular level. When there are higher levels of this hormone during sleep, you tend to experience a more restful night's sleep, helping you to wake up feeling more rested and energized during the day.

You don't have to wait months or even weeks to feel the positive impact of fasting and better sleep. Studies have shown that those who adhered to an IF schedule for just one week saw significant improvement in the quality and quantity of their sleep (Sumeer, 2022).

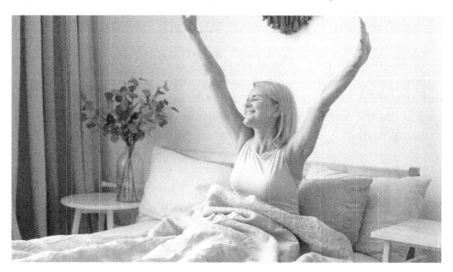

Better Sleep During Menopause

Menopause contributes to various sleep disturbances. Hot flashes can wake you suddenly and keep you tossing and turning throughout the night. Additionally, waking suddenly or frequently throughout the evening can trigger hot flashes, making it difficult to get back to sleep.

Changes in hormone levels can make it harder for the body to slow down at night or cause you to feel more fatigue during the day. Mood changes, higher levels of stress, and overall shifts in your life all disrupt your sleep. Managing your sleep, especially as you get older, is essential for maintaining a healthy life during and after menopause.

Many menopausal women turn to sleep aids, supplements, and other over-the-counter drugs to help them sleep through the night. These aides often provide temporary relief but can cause long-term sleep issues that continue well after menopause. Luckily, there are many natural ways you can gain control over your sleep schedule and feel more rested and energized.

The first thing you want to do is evaluate your bedtime routine. Do you even have a bedtime routine? Many women go hard all day, moving from task to task, wearing many different hats, and eventually crashing into bed at night without giving much thought to a bedtime routine. Intentionally creating a routine helps ease the body into a relaxing state, making it easier to fall asleep and stay asleep.

Your bedtime routine should start two to three hours before your planned bedtime. You want to keep your bedtime the same every night, and it should allow you to get eight hours of sleep every evening. Sticking to the same sleep and wake-up time is essential to regulate the circadian rhythm.

You want to set a time for your last meal during your sleep routine. This can be easy to establish if you're fasting, as it will align with your fasting schedule. You ideally want to have your last "big" meal no later than two hours before your planned bedtime.

You also want to turn off your electronics at least an hour before your planned bedtime. Many studies have shown that the light from electronics, even from your phone, can keep brain activity high, making it harder for it to slow down and let you go to sleep. So instead, read, stretch, journal, meditate, or take a relaxing bath to help unwind and get ready for bed.

You must set up a sleep environment to encourage a more restful night's sleep. Turn the thermostat down, so your bedroom maintains a slightly cooler temperature—68 degrees Fahrenheit tends to be the ideal temperature for most. Ensure you have fans on low to encourage proper air circulation. Wearing comfortable clothes to sleep in will help regulate your body temperature through the night. If necessary, close your blinds to block light, wear a face mask, and turn on a noise machine to drown out distracting sounds.

Establishing a sleep-promoting bedtime routine can lead to a better night's sleep and help you look forward to sleeping more. You can do things throughout the day that can lead to a better night's sleep, such as:

- Don't nap. If you must take a quick snooze during the day, be sure it isn't for longer than 60 minutes. If you must nap, do it earlier in the day.

- Exercise early in the day.

- Cut off your caffeine intake by noon. This means no coffee, chocolates, or any other caffeinated foods or drinks in the later part of the day.

- Avoid alcohol. Not only does it make sleep more difficult, but it can also increase the occurrence of hot flashes.

If your sleep struggles are beyond your control, consider talking to your doctor. There may be other conditions that contribute to your sleep issues. Sleep deprivation is detrimental, and talking with your doctor can lead to effective strategies to improve your sleep and, as a result, improve your overall health.

Insulin is just one of the hormones that intermittent fasting can positively impact. In the next chapter, you'll learn about other hormones that also become harder for the body to manage when we age, which intermittent fasting can help regulate.

Chapter 6:

Balancing Hormones with

Intermittent Fasting

Changes in hormones are expected as you age, which can create issues with your health that feel out of your control. You may be aware of some hormones that are well-known to cause health problems, leading you to believe you need to put a stop to the production of some hormones while boosting others.

No hormone is inherently good or bad. Even cortisol, known as the stress hormone and often viewed in a highly negative manner, helps us maintain normal blood pressure and circulation. It gets a negative reputation because it can lead to "stress" eating.

Estrogen production, which decreases after 40, protects bones and keeps skin moist. Unfortunately, it's also what triggers perimenopause hot flashes.

Every hormone has a benefit and an equal negative side effect. While you may feel like you can't sway the production of these hormones in your body, this, like many other processes, can be managed through healthy habits.

Precaution of Hormonal Imbalance

While fasting provides many health benefits, this doesn't mean it's without its negative impacts. Fasting can cause disruptions in our bodies that can cause you to feel more tired, moody, and struggle with weight management. Does this mean you should avoid fasting? No! Instead, understanding the impacts fasting can have and learning how to combat these effects can lead to having a positive experience with intermittent fasting. First, let's look at the main hormones that can cause extreme fatigue when out of balance.

The Effects of Fasting on Estrogen

Estrogen is the primary female sex hormone that begins to decrease in production as we age. Once we reach menopausal age, estrogen production is significantly depleted, which is why older women struggle more with fatigue and other ailments. An imbalance of estrogen can cause:

- Glucose dysregulation

- Low energy levels

- Weight gain

- Bone density loss

- Muscle mass loss

- Poor skin health

- Poor hair health

- Decrease in cardiovascular health

Estrogen is controlled by the hypothalamic-pituitary-gonadal axis (HPG) and regulates our monthly menstrual cycles. HPG is extremely sensitive, and any body changes can impact the process and production of sex hormones. For instance, metabolic function and higher insulin levels can cause a slowdown of HPG functions, which can trigger the body to go into starvation mode and hold onto fat. Since fasting can cause many of the body's processes to change, this can have a negative impact on estrogen.

The Effects of Fasting on Cortisol

The adrenal glands produce cortisol to regulate body functions, including metabolism, blood pressure, and blood sugar levels. It is released anytime the body is under stress. When you begin intermittent fasting, your body is under extra stress as it becomes accustomed to your new way of eating. An increase in cortisol will increase glucose levels and have a negative impact on insulin production. If cortisol levels remain high for an extended period, you can suffer from adrenal fatigue. Other signs that can indicate you're experiencing higher levels of cortisol in the body include:

- Feeling more anxious or suffering from anxiety.

- Feel less energized despite also feeling high-strung or wired.

- Insomnia or having trouble with sleep.

- Having more sugar or sweet cravings.

The Effects of Fasting on Thyroid Hormones

The thyroid produces specific hormones, T3 and T4, which influence every system and cell found in your body. When you fast, there is a disruption in the balance between the T3 and T4 hormones. An imbalance in thyroid hormones can cause:

- Weight gain

- Anxiety

- Depression

- Dry skin and hair

- Brain fog or forgetfulness

- Irregular cycles

- Inability to regulate body temperature

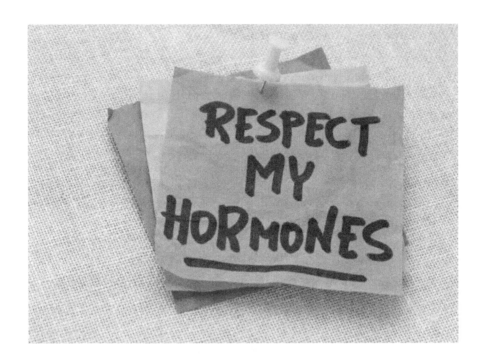

Fasting and Hormones

Although intermittent fasting is relatively straightforward for women, especially those over 50, it requires you to consider the natural hormonal changes your body is going through. Intermittent fasting affects women differently than men, and it isn't for everyone. Intermittent fasting may not work, depending on your current health. It's important to always listen to your body before continuing with intermittent fasting. With this in mind, let's take a closer look at how you can balance your hormones and experience IF benefits.

How Fasting Can Balance Hormones

Intermittent fasting has become highly popular because of its ability to help you lose weight and/or maintain a healthy weight. But it also affects the metabolic systems in the body. The metabolic system is directly connected to the reproductive system in a woman's body, which is why intermittent fasting can significantly impact women's hormonal balance more than men's. The female reproductive system is susceptible to stress. Since fasting causes extra stress in the body, balancing hormones becomes more challenging. However, educating yourself on the effects of fasting will lead to profound positive health effects.

Balancing Insulin

As we covered in the last chapter, intermittent fasting can help control glucose levels by checking our insulin. When we fast for more extended periods, it triggers the fat-burning process of the body. This process keeps insulin levels lower.

Balancing Leptin and Ghrelin

Leptin and ghrelin are hunger hormones. Leptin is a hunger-suppressing hormone that signals to the brain that you're full and the body has enough fuel, so you can stop eating. However, communication with the brain can be damaged, causing the brain not to recognize the leptin signals. As a result, the brain thinks you're starving and triggers hunger signals, so you eat. Ghrelin is the hunger hormone that causes you to feel hungry. Intermittent fasting helps maintain a balance between these two hormones.

Balancing the Human Growth Hormone

The human growth hormone helps the body burn fat as fuel, maintain muscle mass, and keep our bones strong and healthy. Unfortunately, as we age, HGH production decreases, which is why many women struggle more with their weight, loss of muscle mass, and osteoporosis after age 50. Sticking to a fasting schedule can trigger the release of human growth hormone, making it easier to maintain muscle mass and manage weight.

Balancing Cortisol

If you already struggle with chronic stress, it's a good idea to incorporate stress reduction methods into your day before you begin fasting. By gaining control over your stress and lowering your cortisol levels, fasting will have a more positive impact. Slowly transitioning to a fasting schedule is recommended if you have a more stressful lifestyle, such as a demanding job or caring for a sick relative.

Balancing Sex Hormones

Gonadotropin-releasing hormone (GnRH) is the primary hormone that controls the female sex hormones, specifically estrogen and progesterone. It's monitored through the hypothalamic-pituitary-gonadal axis. When women have excess stress, GnRH production is slowed; estrogen and progesterone levels drop.

Estrogen plays a more significant role in the female body outside of reproduction. It provides protective factors for our brain and heart health. It also helps us balance our mood, get better sleep, regulate metabolism, and influences insulin sensitivity. When estrogen levels drop, our health can suffer.

Additionally, the stress your body can experience through prolonged fasting times also impairs the HPG, further slowing reproduction functions. This is why women need to understand the impact fasting can have on the body's systems. However, this doesn't mean that you should avoid fasting. It can provide many benefits when done with a gentle approach and being more aware of what you eat during your eating windows. Including plenty of healthy fats will help balance hormone production.

Balancing Thyroid Hormones

Since fasting affects thyroid hormone, metabolism, and energy usage, you can see improvements in your weight management. This can be accomplished when you provide the right balance of nutrients to your body during your eating window. You don't want to restrict your calorie intake when fasting; you want to provide your body with the most nutritious food options. Sticking to a shorter fasting window can also help keep the thyroid hormones in better balance. Since stress also impairs the conversion of T4 to T3, it's important to prioritize stress management. Getting enough sleep will also help you better balance your thyroid hormones.

Other Effects of Fasting

Intermittent fasting for women requires an individualized approach. Every woman's body may react differently to it. It's important to tune into your body and recognize when fasting is working for you and when it might need to be tweaked. Some key factors to consider when choosing an IF plan are discussed below.

Fasting and Your Menstrual Cycle

Fasting has been shown to benefit women who suffer from PCOS. Those with PCOS often struggle more with their weight and are at greater risk of insulin resistance. Inflammation is also a key contributor to the health problems of those with PCOS. Women with PCOS can benefit from a 16-hour fasting time and see improved symptoms and a more regulated menstrual cycle.

However, women with a regular menstrual cycle may see their periods become unregulated when fasting for 16 or more hours. This is due to the disruption that fasting can have on the luteinizing hormone, which is responsible for keeping the ovaries on a regular schedule. The luteinizing hormone is affected by GnRH, which will halt reproduction hormones when under stress, resulting in an irregular period.

If your cycle is already regular, you want to stick with a shorter fasting window. It's also important not to restrict your calorie intake. Longer fasting times and excessive calorie restrictions can significantly disrupt female hormone production.

Fasting for Premenopausal, Menopausal, and Postmenopausal Women

Those who are nearing menopause or are of premenopausal age may benefit more from intermittent fasting. The main concern for women and fasting is its impact on estrogen levels. However, estrogen production nearly ceases in the female body as we age. Any concern or negative impact that intermittent fasting has on estrogen is less concerning because it provides substantial benefits in other areas of health negatively impacted by lower estrogen levels. For instance, low estrogen increases the risk of insulin resistance, heart disease, cardiovascular disease, and poor brain health. Fasting can help reduce these risks and manage your weight, lowering your risk of serious health complications. Postmenopausal women may additionally benefit from intermittent fasting, and many believe that older women can have more success with it since their hormonal balance becomes more stable at this point.

Fasting and Your Sex Drive

Most studies around sex hormonal balance are focused on men. In one such study, men who adhered to a longer fast saw decreased sexual desire. This may—or may not—be true for women. If fasting causes you to be more moody and low on energy, it's understandable why you may not be interested in sex. However, intermittent fasting should have the reverse effect, leaving you feeling more energized and in a better mood. And since it helps manage weight, you may feel more confident and attractive. This can increase your sex drive!

When to Stop Intermittent Fasting

Intermittent fasting provides many health benefits, but if you already struggle with hormonal imbalance, it might not be the best fit for you. You should stop if you experience hormonal imbalance symptoms that worsen when you fast. If you aren't sure if you struggle with hormone production, some clear signs to watch out for include:

- Your period stops, or you experience irregular periods when they were regular before you started fasting.

- You're having more difficulty falling asleep or staying asleep through the night.

- You notice changes in your digestion. For instance, you feel more bloated after eating or have an upset stomach.

- There is a shift in your metabolism, or you feel more drained and less energetic throughout the day.

- You start to have cognitive issues, like brain fog or an increase in forgetfulness.

- You notice changes in your moods.

- You see negative changes in your hair and skin.

- You suddenly can't get warm and always feel cold.

You can take certain preventive measures to help avoid these adverse effects while fasting. For example, not fasting on consecutive days, shortening your fasting window to 12 to 14 hours, drinking more water, and easing into longer fasting windows can help you successfully transition to intermittent fasting.

Additionally, if you have shortened your fasting window and taken other preventive measures to combat adverse effects, you should reconsider what you eat. Yes, certain foods can also impact your hormone production. If you're experiencing any clear signs of hormonal imbalance or negative effects of fasting, try eliminating or reducing your intake of the following foods.

Red Meats

Fatty meats or those high in saturated fats can spike estrogen production and disrupt other hormonal balances. Swapping out red meat for eggs or fatty fish helps regulate hormone production and provides additional health-boosting properties.

Soy

While soy can help menopausal women combat the effect of hot flashes, it can also disrupt the female reproductive system. It's because soy contains phytoestrogen and responds the same in the body as estrogen does when consumed. This can lead to irregular cycles and negative consequences on your hormonal balance and reproductive health.

Dairy

While dairy products, like milk, can provide the body with essential nutrients in small amounts, they can wreak havoc on your hormones when consumed in higher amounts. Milk contains natural sugars, which can throw off gut health and increase inflammation. It can also increase triglyceride levels and negatively impact insulin levels. As a result, this can lead to various hormonal imbalances.

Caffeine

Your cup or two of coffee a day can be an underlying culprit to your hormonal struggles. Caffeine increases cortisol, the stress hormone, and as you now know, stress disrupts hormone production in many ways. So while you might need the cup of Joe to wake you up and keep you alert in the morning, it can make it more challenging for you to maintain a healthy lifestyle.

Processed Foods

It should be no surprise that processed foods deteriorate your health on many levels. They contain high amounts of sugar, sodium, and preservatives, increasing inflammation. These ingredients also negatively affect the adrenal glands, which oversee most hormone production in the body.

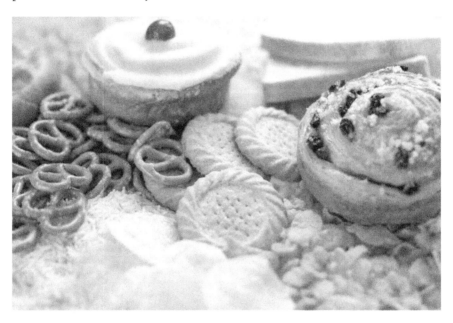

Excess Vegetables

Let me first say that this isn't a problem with all vegetables. You should and can eat most vegetables freely without concern. However, there are a few vegetables that you want to limit if you're struggling with hormonal balance. Cruciferous vegetables—broccoli, cauliflower, and kale—can disrupt functions of the thyroid gland when consumed in high quantities. Other vegetables, like potatoes, tomatoes, eggplant, and peppers, should be eaten in smaller amounts. While these vegetables provide many nutrients, they can increase inflammation, throwing your hormones out of sync. You don't need to eliminate these few vegetables completely but do eat them more sparingly than others.

We have covered various topics that revolve around what you eat. Are you feeling more confident about taking control of your health in your 50s and beyond? Now, it's time to cover a topic that most women over 50 think they need to avoid: exercise.

Chapter 7:

How Exercise Can Lower Blood Sugar, Reduce Inflammation, and Improve Gut Health

How much do you need to exercise to experience the most health benefits? Thirty minutes? An hour?

Just 20 minutes of exercise can act as an anti-inflammatory, boost your immune system, help you lose weight, and improve your mood.

You may think, "I haven't exercised in years, and now I'm too old to start again." Whatever negative beliefs you have about exercising as you get older should be pushed aside. It doesn't matter what age you are. Starting an exercise routine is an essential component to better health.

Exercise When You're Over 50

We need to discuss exercise because it's crucial to a healthy lifestyle. However, we discussed many dieting aspects of maintaining optimal health because even with exercise, you can't out-exercise a bad diet. You can exercise intently every day, but if you aren't eating the right foods to nourish your body, exercise isn't going to help improve your health.

Exercise does more than helps you lose weight and look great at any age. Maintaining an active lifestyle, 50 and beyond, is a big part of properly taking care of yourself. Even if you haven't exercised much in your earlier years, it's never too late to get active and take advantage of all its benefits.

Improving and maintaining muscle mass over 50 is a major concern for women. It's common that the average woman will experience a 1% loss of muscle mass yearly after the age of 50 (The Y, 2019). Due to fluctuations in hormone production, it can be hard to feel as physically strong as you once did. In connection with muscle mass, bone density and strength also becomes problematic. Exercising can help maintain muscle mass and bone density, keeping you at a lower risk of becoming overweight or having osteoporosis.

How fat is disrupted or stored in the body after 50 also changes, putting older women at a greater risk of severe health problems. Once menopause hits, the body begins storing more fat around the abdomen, which can put pressure on the vital organs. Regular exercise can help you eliminate this stored fat and keep your internal process clear of distributions.

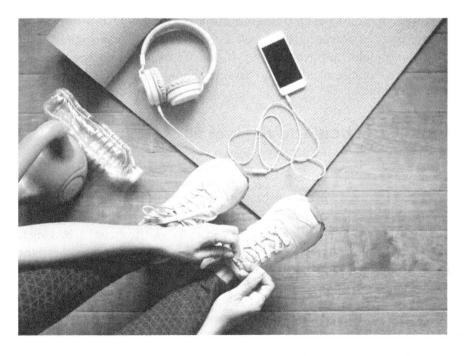

Types of Exercise

Exercise should be fun and beneficial, but many view it as an obligation or punishment. Understanding and creating a fitness routine that's best for you and your health goals can feel overwhelming. No clear exercise regime will work for everyone, but incorporating a few key varieties of physical activity can help you stay fit and healthy through menopause and beyond.

Strength Training for Women Over 50

Many women shy away from strength training because they initially think that lifting weights will result in bulking up or increase their risk of injury. Strength training isn't just about lifting weights. Resistance training, using your body weight, exercise bands, or medicine balls, can also be used in strength training.

There are also plenty of groups or classes you can join to help you increase your muscle mass. Search social media for exercise groups, see what classes your local gym offers, or find your nearest YMCA or recreation center to find various programs you can participate in. If group sessions don't interest you, you can easily perform a strength training routine in your home with little to no additional equipment. Give the following strength training exercises a try.

Planks

Planks are a versatile exercise that uses your body weight to strengthen the whole body. Since they focus on developing the core and lower back muscles, they're also ideal for improving balance.

Low planks can be beneficial if you're getting into an exercise routine. For a low-plank lie on the floor on your stomach. Bend your arms so your elbows are positioned under your shoulder, and your hands should be below your forehead; they can be pressed palm-side down on the ground or clenched in a loose fist. Now, with your feet about hip-width apart, pop up on your toes. Engage your core, meaning you want to tighten the abdominal muscles as you lift your hips off the ground. You want to create a straight line with your body from your head to your toes.

Hold this position for 30 seconds. Keep your weight distributed between your forearms and toes. If your back starts to dip, re-engage your core by tightening your abdomen, glute, and quad muscles. Be mindful not to strain your neck. Keep your eyes focused on your hands. Don't let your shoulders round as you hold yourself up. Your shoulder blades should be pulled toward the midline of your back, not stretched apart. If you feel more of your weight is supported by your shoulders, adjust so you bring them together to keep your weight distributed throughout the body.

Additionally, don't hold your breath as you keep your plank pose. You want to take deep, long breaths as you plank.

If you want to challenge yourself, you can shift your plank position to a higher one. This is the same as a low plank, except instead of staying on your forearms, you'll push yourself up higher so your arms are straight and you're holding yourself up with just your hands. A high plank is simply a push-up where you pause in the up position. Keep your hands a little more than shoulder-width apart, and don't lock your elbows when you push yourself up. As you hold the high plank, the same rules apply as if you're doing a low plank. Keep your body weight distributed throughout the body and keep your hips in a straight line.

Chair squats

Chair squats are great for toning your lower body, but they also help improve your balance. You'll want a chair as you begin to get used to the movements of this exercise.

Essentially, this exercise will mimic how you sit in a chair, but instead of sitting, you pause and then stand. Start by standing in front of a chair with your feet about hip-width apart. Point your toes out slightly; this is important because you want your knees to align in the same direction as your toes when you lift yourself back up. You don't want your knees to drive inward toward each other.

When ready, distribute your weight evenly throughout your feet. Take a deep breath, and on the exhale, lower your butt to the chair. You can keep your hands on your hips, crossed over your chest, so your hands touch your shoulders, or stretch your arms out in front of your body for extra balance support. Lowering to the chair, lean your torso forward while keeping your back straight. This may feel awkward initially, as we often try to keep our torso straight when sitting. Lean from the hips as your back lowers to the chair. Once you're a few inches from the chair seat, pause for three seconds, then slowly lift yourself back up to your standing position. Repeat at least five times.

Chest Fly

For this exercise, you'll need a set of hand weights. A filled water bottle, canned food, or even bags of beans can be a great substitute for traditional hand weights. Just be sure you're using the same amount of weight in each hand.

To begin, lay on your back on the floor. Laying on an exercise mat can be more comfortable but isn't necessary. Bend your knees, so your feet are also flat on the floor. Take a weight in each hand and stretch your arms to your sides with your palms facing up. Exhale as you lift your arms above your chest, bringing your palms together. Inhale and lower your arms back to the floor. Repeat five to ten times.

Yoga

Yoga combines all the exercises you should be doing in one session. Many people think yoga is a meditative or deep-breathing movement routine. Still, it also incorporates strength training using your body weight, stretching, and balance, and it can even be a great cardio exercise, depending on which type you do.

Stretching is vital to keep your body flexible and also helps keep your mind flexible. Yoga further enhances your mind and body flexibility. Many yoga poses also improve your balance, such as standing on one foot or shifting from standing to floor poses.

There are various types of yoga you can try. You can find yoga sequences focusing on flexibility, better sleep, weight loss, stress reduction, and many others. You can also find a few yoga poses to help keep your body stretched and energized throughout the day. You can join a yoga class at your local yoga studio or gym or find a yoga video online that focuses on your specific needs.

Remember that while yoga is a prime example of how you incorporate different types of exercise into one routine, this is true for many kinds of exercise. For example, walking stretches and strengthens the leg muscles while trimming your waist. You also stretch your body and work on your balance when you lift weights.

How Much Exercise Do You Need?

No matter your age, doctors recommend the same amount of exercise for all adults to be around 150 minutes, which averages out to 30 minutes five days a week. This time gets cut in half to just 75 minutes if you focus on vigorous activity every week. However, getting the right mix of different exercise types in those minutes does make a difference.

Before you jump into any exercise routine, it is important that you speak with your doctor first. Not only will this reassure you that you're in the best current health to increase your physical activity, but it can also help you find the best exercise routine to reach your health goals.

After getting the thumbs-up from your doctor, you want to create an exercise routine that fits your lifestyle and one that you can commit to for the long term. As you're creating your exercise plan, keep the following in mind:

- You want most of your exercise time composed of aerobic or cardio activities. If you can't fit a 30-minute aerobic activity into your schedule, it can be completed in three 10-minute sessions. For instance, you can go for a 10-minute walk in the morning, afternoon, and evening. During these 10 minutes, you should get your heart rate up and breathe more deeply. Aerobic exercises include swimming, biking, walking or jogging, or dancing.

- Twice a week, you should focus on strength training activities. Remember, strength training can include resistance training. If you prefer to walk as your primary exercise, find a hill to walk up or add a set of weights to mix in resistance training.

- If you begin to experience issues with balance, which is also quite common for older women, adding balancing exercise three days a week will help you improve your balance and mobility.

- Find a group or class to join once a week. Group programs can keep you motivated and help you enjoy your workout more. You can find many types of groups or classes in your area. From kickboxing and dance classes to strength training and running groups, your local gym will likely offer various classes. You can also search social media to find local running groups for women, including menopausal, moms, and over 50 groups.

The Connection Between Blood Sugar and Exercise

Exercise greatly influences blood sugar levels and can help improve insulin sensitivity. Performing just 15 minutes of light to moderate exercise after you eat can help keep blood sugar levels lower (Byrne, 2021). Exercising contracts the muscle, allowing the cells in the body to take in more glucose, whether there is insulin flowing in the bloodstream. In the short term, this can help lower blood sugar levels. In the long term, regular physical activity can help lower A1C, which measures your blood sugar levels over three months. While it's important to keep daily blood sugar levels lower, it's just as important to understand how your blood sugar levels change over time. Unlike blood sugar levels measured in milligrams per deciliter (mg/dL), A1C is expressed as a percentage.

What A1C reveals is how many of your red blood cells, which carry oxygen throughout the body, have sugar molecules attached to them. A healthy person will have an A1C below 5.7%. Those in the prediabetes category tend to have a percentage between 5.7% to 6.4%. Those who have diabetes or are at the greatest risk of developing diabetes have an A1C above 6.5%.

Exercise and Diabetes

Exercise is essential to diabetes management, but some precautions must be considered. Those on insulin or diabetes medication are often at greater risk of hypoglycemia. Adjusting your insulin or carbohydrate intake can reduce this risk.

Before you begin an exercise routine, you need to speak with your doctor to understand your risk of hypoglycemia. Your health care team will provide you with the best approach to incorporating physical activity into your daily routine while safely managing and lowering your blood sugar levels.

Wait to exercise until after you check your blood sugar levels. This is important as exercise will lower your blood sugar levels, and you want to prevent them from dropping too low. If your blood sugar does drop too low during or after your exercise routine, you want to treat it immediately. You can refer to the 15-15 rule outlined below to help manage blood sugar levels during or after exercise.

The 15-15 Rule

First, check your blood sugar. If your levels are below 100 mg/dL, consume 15 grams of carbs to raise the levels. Fifteen grams of carbs equal:

- ½ cup of juice or 4 ounces of juice
- 1 tablespoon of honey
- 1 glucose gel tube
- 4 glucose tablets

Wait 15 minutes, then recheck your blood sugar. If your levels are still below 100, consume another 15 grams of carbs. Repeat this process until your blood sugar levels reach at least 100 mg/dL.

If you're mid-exercise when experiencing low blood sugar symptoms, you'll need to pause your workout until you raise your sugar levels. You can continue your workout after your blood sugar levels have reached a safe level, but you'll need to monitor them closely throughout the rest of your workout. Remember that blood sugar levels can continue to decrease well after you have stopped exercising, so it's important to check your levels throughout the day. If you frequently experience hypoglycemia while exercising, you want to speak with your doctor to help formulate the best exercise plan to manage your sugar levels safely.

Exercise as an Anti-Inflammatory

Inflammation contributes to diabetes, cardiovascular disease, a decline in brain cognition, and many other chronic conditions. Exercise can help improve the body's inflammatory response and alleviate inflammation. Research has shown that just 20 minutes of moderate and even low-intensity exercise can help reduce inflammation (Brubaker, 2017).

The most effective types of exercise that can help you reduce inflammation include:

- Yoga or any deep-breathing exercise that incorporates gentle movements.

- Bodyweight exercises or resistant-type exercises, such as planks, squats, and push-ups.

- Mobility exercises, such as self-myofascial release exercises and foam roller exercises. These are often massage-based movements or pressure-applied exercises that improve the range of motion and muscle function.

- Cycling can be highly beneficial for older women, whether you're riding your 10-speed outside in nice weather or joining a cycling class. This exercise is easy on your joints while also helping improve your range of motion and reduce inflammation.

Exercises to Improve Gut Health

Exercising can alter the gut microbiome. As you've learned, the right balance of gut bacteria is crucial for keeping the body functioning at its best. A small study at the University of Illinois shows how exercise can positively impact the gut microbiome in just six weeks. This study included 32 participants, 18 who were considered lean and 14 who were considered obese. Each participant's gut microbiome was sampled before they were placed on a cardiovascular exercise routine: working out 30 to 60 minutes three times a week for six weeks. After six weeks, their gut microbiome was sampled again. Researchers found that many participants had an increase in specific gut bacteria that produce short-chain fatty acids, which are known to reduce inflammation and help reduce the risk of heart disease and diabetes (Pratt, 2018).

Once participants returned to their everyday lifestyles, their gut microbiome returned to how it was before their six-week exercise program. This study indicates that regular exercise can benefit gut health. Aside from cardio-based exercise programs, walking, cycling, stomach crunches, sit-ups, and other abdominal-strengthening exercises benefit gut health.

It is important to note that regular exercise is the key to maintaining gut health. Exercising for a few weeks or months and then returning to a sedentary or lower physical activity level will cause your gut health to revert to how it was before you started exercising. As with many other lifestyle changes, if you want to experience the benefits for the long term, you must make a change for the long term.

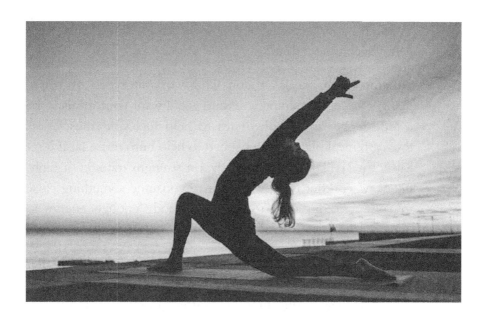

How to Exercise Safely While Fasting

While there are many benefits to fasting and exercising, combining the two can have a downside. When you're fasting, your body naturally will turn on its fat-burning process. However, exercising while fasting can cause the body to turn to the muscles for fuel. You may also find that you don't have as much endurance or perform at your peak when fasting and exercising simultaneously. In the long term, you can end up depleting your body of the calories it needs to provide your body with enough energy, and as a result, this can cause your metabolism to slow down.

This doesn't mean you have to choose one or the other. You can still adhere to a fasting plan while also getting the exercise you need. To help you create the most effective IF exercise plan for your lifestyle, consider the following:

- Plan your fasting and exercise times. This can take some trial and error. You may start exercising before your fasting window but don't have the energy or stamina you usually have.

Switching your exercise during your eating window can be a better accommodation.

- Structure your meals around your workout types. If you're doing a strength training workout, you'll want your meals to be a little higher in carbohydrates to help fuel your muscles. A low-carb meal plan is better suited to help burn more fat if it's a cardio or HIIT day. Additionally, on strength training or high-intensity workout days, you want to consume something close to your workout time to give your body enough energy to power through your workout.

- Incorporate muscle-building foods after workouts. Whether working out during your feeding window or before your fasting time, you want your first meal after your workout to help maintain your muscle mass. Lean proteins, healthy fats, and complex carbs are essential. You want to consume more lean proteins and healthy fats to help regenerate your muscle mass.

- If you're doing a 24-hour fast, choose low-intensity workouts, like gentle yoga or walking, on your fasting days.

- No matter what IF plan you're following, stay adequately hydrated. When fasting, you should try to consume more water. Also, be mindful of replenishing your electrolytes. While most electrolyte drinks contain calories and shouldn't be consumed during your fasting window, you want to ensure you take some electrolytes when you exercise.

Always listen to your body. You can try all the above suggestions, but if you're feeling weak, dizzy, or not yourself, this is a red flag that your fast or exercise regime isn't right for you. Please don't ignore these signs, as they can indicate something more severe or have adverse side effects.

In the next chapter, you'll learn a variety of additional tips and tricks that will make eating right, fasting, exercising, and shifting to a healthy lifestyle an easy transition.

Chapter 8:

Intermittent Fasting Hacks—

Making Your Lifestyle Easier

How do you turn everything you've learned into a lifestyle that's easy to commit to? Simple adjustments, like eating a protein-packed diet while intermittent fasting, can lead to more fat loss than a standard heart-healthy diet (Landsverk, 2021). Learning to incorporate all this information can seem like a lot to do all at once. However, making just a few simple changes that combine the techniques previously discussed will minimize the effort and resistance to making the necessary health changes that'll improve your health and happiness.

Eight IF Hacks

Transitioning to an IF plan doesn't have to be overwhelming. The great thing about intermittent fasting is that, for most people, the majority of your fasting window will take place while you sleep. However, there are a few other great tricks you can use that will lead to greater success while fasting to help you lose weight and improve your overall health.

Keep Your Meals Balanced

It can be challenging to eat healthy meals, especially that first meal after your fasting window. Until you get used to allowing yourself to be hungry for a little bit—remember you shouldn't feel like you're starving—you might be tempted to reach for whatever you can to curb the hunger. Many people have this misconception that they can eat whatever they want if they stick to an IF plan, but it's more important to consume whole foods. You want meals to provide you with essential vitamins and minerals, so you stay full for longer, feel more energized, and keep your body fueled while fasting.

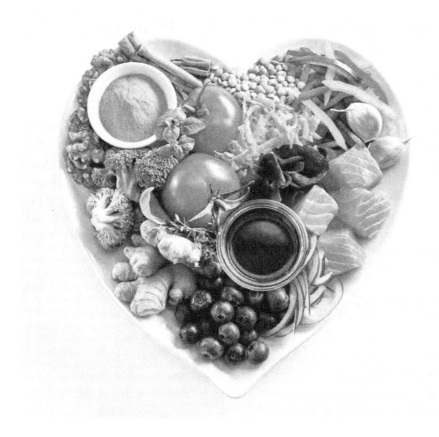

Don't Accidentally Break Your Fast

If the first thing you reach for in the morning is a cup of coffee with cream and sugar, a diet soda, or a cup of juice, you want to reconsider these options. Each of these will break your fast. If you have one or two hours left in your fasting window, this will defeat the purpose of fasting and minimize the benefits. Even if you choose a low-sugar beverage, many will contain artificial sweeteners, stimulating your appetite. Not only will you break your fast early, but you'll also be more likely to overeat throughout the day. Instead, reach for a cup of tea, black coffee, or water for your early mornings.

Remember Fasting Means No Eating

Fasting means not eating food, not even a small piece of chocolate or fruit. This is important, as even consuming a small amount of food will trigger insulin release, shifting the body from burning fat to storing fat. Additionally, breaking your fast before your body has gotten used to the IF plan can result in it going into starvation mode. You'll store more fat instead of losing it. For your plan to work, you must choose a fasting window that works for your schedule and commit to it. If an 18-hour window often results in you sneaking in something small in the middle of your fast, you want to choose a shorter fasting window.

Hydration Is Essential

You want to increase the amount of water you drink throughout your day. Staying hydrated while trying to lose weight or improve your health is key to success. Drinking a glass of water before meals can help combat hunger and reduce the risk of overeating. If you need to liven up your water, you can always add slices of fresh fruit or herbs for more flavor.

Fill Your Fasting Window with Activities

While most of your fasting window will often be spent sleeping, you'll still have a few hours where you'll need to keep yourself busy, so you don't succumb to the temptation to eat. Having a solid evening and morning routine can help you get through those hours of your fasting window. Consider going for a walk in the evening, reading, or running errands. In the morning, add in some meditation, reading, or journaling. Keeping yourself busy will help you distract your thoughts from eating to something more productive.

Get Your Full Eight Hours of Sleep

You may need to get more than eight hours of sleep, but you want to ensure that you get at least eight hours every night. Sleep is essential for repairing the body. Getting the right amount of sleep will help regulate and improve your metabolism. Adjust your bedtime for eight hours if you need to be up at a specific time. For instance, if you need to be up at 6 a.m., you must get to sleep by 10 p.m. This doesn't mean you crawl into bed at 10 p.m. as you most likely aren't going to fall asleep as soon as you hit the bed, but you're ready to turn the lights off at 10 p.m.

Creating a solid evening routine can help you get into the habit of getting to bed at the correct time. Your evening should consist of relaxing and enjoyable activities. Reading, stretching, taking a warm shower, getting things ready for the next day, and anything that doesn't stimulate the brain too much is a suitable activity. You want to avoid anything that requires using an electronic device; even an ereader can stimulate brain activity, making it harder to get to sleep.

If you aren't used to sleeping early, ease into an earlier bedtime. Get to bed just 15 minutes earlier. If you often find yourself up until midnight, make your bedtime 11:45. Do this for a few days, then move to another 15 minutes earlier. Continue to do this until you have reached your ideal bedtime.

Manage Your Stress

When you experience high stress levels, it can be impossible to stick with an IF plan. Stress will cause you to feel more hungry and crave more unhealthy foods. Having a few stress management routines in place will help you minimize stress, combat the desire to eat unhealthy food, and will also help you sleep better. Begin reducing your stress with activities like guided meditation, going outdoors, journaling, etc. Ironically, these activities significantly add to your evening or morning routine.

Add in Exercise

Exercise is what will ramp up your weight loss success. While fasting, you need to take caution in the type of exercise you do, depending on the length of your fasting window. This doesn't mean you need to avoid exercise. Adding an exercise routine to your day will help you retain higher energy levels, sleep better, reduce stress, and help you maintain your muscle mass. Remember that to get the most benefits, you should incorporate a few different exercises, including cardio and strength training.

The Mediterranean Diet

Research has shown that a Mediterranean diet, as discussed earlier in this book, can help lower inflammation by beneficially altering gut bacteria. A 2020 study noted the difference between the gut bacteria of people who switched to a Mediterranean diet and those who ate a typical diet. Those on the Mediterranean diet saw changes in the gut microbiome linked to reduced risk of certain cancers, insulin resistance, cell damage, and fatty liver disease, among other conditions. These severe health ailments are often a result of an unbalanced gut microbiome. More significant about this study was that once the research was over and individuals on the Mediterranean diet returned to their previous eating patterns, changes in their gut bacteria also reverted to previous states (Harvard Health Publishing, 2020). This is important because if you want lasting beneficial results, you must make dietary changes and accept a new way of living. Creating new habits is not just something you do to help you lose weight, but something you do for overall better health for the rest of your life.

Another study at the University Medical Center Groningen, located in the Netherlands, uncovered how the Mediterranean diet could reduce inflammation. This study included participants with various inflammatory conditions, like Crohn's disease, ulcerative colitis, and irritable bowel syndrome. Included were participants who didn't suffer from any inflammatory condition and consumed either a

Mediterranean-style diet or one higher in red meats, refined sugar, and fast foods. Individuals who ate Mediterranean meals had an increase in beneficial bacteria growth and a decrease in inflammatory marker levels. Those on the traditional diet plan showed the opposite: higher growth of unhelpful gut bacteria and more elevated inflammation markers (Grey, 2019).

Both studies reinforce the benefits of switching to and sticking with a plant-based diet. You can further enhance the benefits of the Mediterranean diet by incorporating an intermittent fasting plan.

Intermittent Fasting and the Mediterranean Diet

Intermittent fasting and combination with the Mediterranean diet can help you streamline your weight-loss efforts and lead you to better health. Since the Mediterranean diet already focuses on healthy, wholesome, and nutritious foods, it only makes sense that combining it with the benefits of intermittent fasting is an ideal pairing. Some tips for ensuring success while fasting and transitioning to the Mediterranean diet include:

- Use extra-virgin olive oil (EVOO) as your primary source of healthy fats. The Mediterranean diet encourages using EVOO frequently, so be sure you're using the highest quality EVOO and use it for non-cooking purposes. Mixing it with herbs, fruit juices, or different kinds of vinegar is a healthy way to create salad dressing and dipping sauces.

- Use fish and plant-based protein, like lentils and beans, as your primary source of protein. Remember that when fasting, you want your first meal after your fasting window to include lean proteins to help fuel your muscles and brain functions and keep you full longer. The Mediterranean diet encourages eating plenty of lean fatty fish, like salmon and tuna.

- Use herbs and spices more than you use salt. They will keep your food full of flavor. If you only eat unseasoned vegetables and meals, they will get boring quickly. Additionally, many spices and herbs, like turmeric and ginger, provide additional nutrients to boost your health.

- Keep your meals more plant-based with a mix of fruits, vegetables, and whole grains. Oats mixed with berries are a fiber-rich breakfast option to start your day healthfully. Aim to eat green leafy vegetables at least daily as part of a salad or a sauteed vegetable side dish.

When choosing the best IF plan to pair with the Mediterranean diet, most time-restricted plans—18:6, 16:8, or 14:10—are ideal over 24-hour fasts. Remember, tune into what your body is telling you. If a longer fasting window leaves you feeling like you're starving, unable to focus, or moody, shorten your fasting window.

Mediterranean Diet 14-Day Meal Plan

All meals with an asterisk (*) near them can be found in the bonus recipe chapter.

Week 1

Monday
- **Breakfast**: 2 eggs cooked as you prefer with whole grain toast and a banana
- **Snack:** Greek yogurt with blueberries and nuts
- **Lunch:** *Cobb salad
- **Snack:** An apple
- **Dinner:** White bean soup

Tuesday
- **Breakfast:** *Berry crisp
- **Snack:** Roasted chickpeas

- **Lunch:** Leftover white bean soup and a piece of fruit
- **Snack:** Raw vegetables and hummus
- **Dinner:** *Sheet pan chicken and vegetables

Wednesday
- **Breakfast:** *Blueberry breakfast oats
- **Snack:** ¼ cup almonds
- **Lunch:** Turkey lettuce wrap and a cup of lentil soup
- **Snack:** Raw vegetables and hummus
- **Dinner:** Grilled fish and vegetables

Thursday
- **Breakfast:** *Almond green smoothie bowl
- **Snack:** Olives and feta cheese
- **Lunch:** Leftover sheet pan chicken and vegetables with pita bread
- **Snack:** Whole grain crackers and cheese
- **Dinner:** *Sweet potatoes curry

Friday
- **Breakfast:** Leftover berry crisp
- **Snack:** Piece of fruit
- **Lunch:** *Avocado quesadillas
- **Snack:** Olives and cheese
- **Dinner:** Grilled chicken and vegetables skewer

Saturday
- **Breakfast:** *Almond green smoothie bowl
- **Snack:** Handful of mixed nuts
- **Lunch:** Leftover sweet potato curry
- **Snack:** Raw vegetables and hummus
- **Dinner:** *Chicken-zucchini noodle bowl

Sunday

- **Breakfast:** 2 eggs with sauteed spinach and an orange
- **Snack:** Mixed nuts and dried apricots
- **Lunch:** *Shrimp lettuce wraps
- **Snack:** A piece of fruit
- **Dinner:** *Black bean soup

Week 2

Monday

- **Breakfast:** *Pumpkin pie oats
- **Snack:** Roasted chickpeas
- **Lunch:** Leftover black bean soup
- **Snack:** Cheese and whole wheat crackers
- **Dinner:** *Mediterranean chicken with avocado tapenade

Tuesday

- **Breakfast:** *Berry peach smoothie bowl
- **Snack:** Mini sweet peppers with hummus
- **Lunch:** Tuna salad over mixed greens and vegetables
- **Snack:** Piece of fruit
- **Dinner:** *Vegan tacos with pickled onions

Wednesday

- **Breakfast:** *Pumpkin pie oats
- **Snack:** Greek yogurt with fresh berries
- **Lunch:** Mixed salad and small soup.
- **Snack:** Nuts and a small piece of dark chocolate
- **Dinner:** *Spicy egg and tomato sauce skillet

Thursday

- **Breakfast:** *Blueberry breakfast oats

- **Snack:** Apple and nut butter
- **Lunch:** *Shrimp lettuce wraps
- **Snack:** Raw vegetables and hummus
- **Dinner:** *Mediterranean salad with quinoa and millet

Friday
- **Breakfast:** Two eggs, whole grain toast, and a piece of fruit
- **Snack:** Greek yogurt with fresh berries
- **Lunch:** Leftover Mediterranean salad
- **Snack:** Handful of nuts
- **Dinner:** *Sesame chicken shredded veggie bowl

Saturday
- **Breakfast:** *Tofu scramble
- **Snack:** Apple slices and nut butter
- **Lunch:** Leftover sesame chicken shredded veggie bowl
- **Snack:** Sliced cheese, olive, and whole grain crackers
- **Dinner:** *Grilled salmon with lemon and roasted vegetables

Sunday
- **Breakfast:** *Blueberry breakfast oats
- **Snack:** Greek yogurt and berries
- **Lunch:** Leftover salmon
- **Snack:** Raw vegetables and hummus
- **Dinner:** Vegetable stew

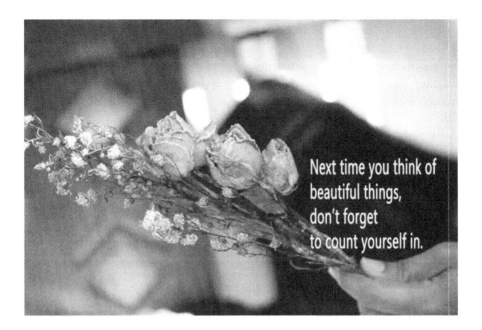

Next time you think of beautiful things, don't forget to count yourself in.

Affirmation to Inspire

What does affirmation have to do with living a healthy lifestyle? Getting older can often leave you feeling uncertain, insecure, and not as confident as you once were. Reminding yourself of the beautiful, fierce, and vibrant woman you are will help boost your confidence.

Affirmations can be a powerful tool that helps you maintain a positive mindset and outlook on your body and health. Repeating a positive affirmation daily can help combat stress, increase motivation, and make healthier choices (Moore, 2019). This is based on neuroscience research that shows repeating positive phrases can rewire the way your brain processes thoughts. When your thoughts change, your behaviors change.

This is a simple and effortless habit you can fit into your day multiple times a day. Choose a phrase that challenges a limiting belief or negative thought about yourself. When you begin to shift from negative to positive, your brain will automatically begin to seek evidence to support those thoughts. This is a useful practice when adopting new healthy habits you might struggle to stick with. Repeating an affirmation helps support the changes you desire. They can lead to making nutritional choices, going for that run in the morning, or meditating before bed.

As simple as the practice is, it's just as easy not to do, which is why many don't repeat these positive phrases daily. Be aware that what we believe becomes our reality whether we think positively or negatively. Consistency and being genuine when you repeat these phrases are the keys to making affirmations work.

Choose one phrase, look at yourself in the mirror, and repeat the phrase. You can repeat it as many times as you need, and you can do this at any time during your day. Repeating the phrase three to five times often has the most benefit. To help get started, you can read over the affirmations below. Choose one or two to begin with.

- *I accept the process of aging and acknowledge the benefits that maturity can bring.*
- *I become wiser, more patient, and more tolerant as I age.*
- *My mind is sharper than ever before.*
- *I may be slowing down, but I am growing stronger.*
- *I feel capable of handling any situation that comes along.*
- *I am a better listener because I learn to listen to my inner voice.*
- *I learn how to respond to a whole variety of thoughts with kindness.*
- *I am conscious of my feelings. I am aware of my pain and suffering.*
- *I make a choice to allow myself to feel better each day.*
- *I choose to let go of fear which causes stress, which leads to illness.*
- *I release my fears, and begin to heal and grow healthier.*
- *I believe that the beauty of life is in the choices and intentions we live by.*
- *I can choose to live fully and welcome all that life offers.*
- *I choose to age gracefully. I enjoy the process of living.*
- *I am grateful for my experiences so far and thankful for my blessings.*
- *I am thankful for the gift of life.*
- *As I grow older, I learn how to love and accept myself.*
- *I choose to be joyful as I age.*

- *I choose to love myself.*
- *I am worthy and deserving of love, respect, and happiness.*
- *I am confident in my abilities and experience.*
- *I am proud of my life achievements and am excited for new opportunities.*
- *I am strong, capable, and resilient.*
- *I embrace my age and all its gifts and challenges.*
- *I am grateful for my life and all its richness and joy*
- *I choose to enjoy each moment of my journey today.*

You can take control of your thoughts and feelings by practicing positive affirmations instead of focusing on negative thoughts. By consciously focusing on positive thoughts and affirmations, you create a more positive outlook on life. This can have lasting effects on your mental health and well-being, as it helps to reduce stress levels, improve mood, increase self-esteem and confidence, and promote healthy relationships. Positive thinking is a powerful tool for personal growth that everyone should use to their advantage!

Chapter 9:

Bonus Recipes!

I wouldn't give you all this information and introduce you to the best diet and eating plan without adding some delicious recipes! You'll find that creating healthy meals shouldn't scare you, even if you aren't a master in the kitchen.

20-Minute Recipes

Blueberry Breakfast Oats

Servings: 1 mug muffin

Prep and cook time: 5 minutes

Ingredients:

- 2 tsp. coconut oil
- ¼ cup blueberries
- ¼ cup whole-wheat pastry flour
- 1 tbsp. rolled oats
- ½ tsp. cinnamon
- ¼ tsp. baking powder
- ¼ cup unsweetened almond or oat milk
- 1 tbsp. coconut sugar
- ¼ tsp. pure vanilla extract
- 2 tsp. toasted pecans (chopped)
- ¼ tsp. sea salt

Directions:

1. Stir the flour, oats, cinnamon, baking powder, sugar, and salt in a small mixing bowl. Set to the side.
2. Whisk the milk, melted coconut oil, and vanilla together in a large 12- or 16-ounce mug.
3. Add half the flour mixture to the mug and mix thoroughly, then add the remaining mixture and stir again.
4. Fold the blueberries into the mug.
5. Place the mug in a microwave and microwave for 1- ½ minutes on high. Keep an eye on the mug and stop if the mixture begins to bubble over the top.
6. When done, the muffin should be slightly firm but moist. If necessary, microwave for another 10 seconds and continue with 10-second intervals until the muffin is cooked all the way through.
7. Allow to cool for a few minutes before eating.

Almond Green Smoothie Bowl

Servings: 2

Prep and cook time: 10 minutes

Ingredients:

- 1 cup Greek yogurt
- 3 tsp. cacao nibs (divided)
- ¼ cup rolled oats
- 1 frozen banana
- ¼ banana (not frozen, sliced)
- ½ cup raspberries
- 2 cups spinach
- 2 tbsp. almond butter
- 2 tbsp. almonds (chopped)

Directions:

1. In a blender, add 2 tsp. cacao nibs, yogurt, almond butter, frozen banana, spinach, and oats. Blend into a puree.
2. Divide the puree between two bowls.
3. Top with the sliced bananas, raspberries, chopped almonds, and the remaining cacao nibs.

Pumpkin Pie Oats

Servings: 2 servings (½ cup each)

Prep and cook time: 5 minutes

Ingredients:

- 2 cups almond milk
- 1 cup water
- 2 ½ cups rolled oats
- ¼ cup pumpkin puree
- 2 tbsp. honey
- 1 tsp. pure vanilla extract
- 1 tsp. ground cinnamon
- ½ tsp. ground nutmeg
- ¼ tsp. all spice
- ¼ tsp. ground cloves
- ¼ tsp. sea salt

Directions:

1. In a small saucepan, bring the water and almond milk to a slight boil over medium heat.
2. Add the remaining ingredients, except the honey, to the saucepan and simmer for 3 minutes. Stir occasionally.
3. Divide the oatmeal between two bowls, drizzle with honey, and enjoy.

Tofu Scramble

Servings: 4

Prep and cook time: 20 minutes

Ingredients:

- 2 tsp. coconut oil
- 16 oz. extra-firm tofu (pressed, drained, pat dry, and crumbled)
- 2 garlic cloves (minced)
- 1 cup red onion (chopped fine)
- 1 cup button mushrooms (chopped)
- 1 cup baby spinach
- ¼ cup nutritional yeast
- 2 tsp. turmeric
- 2 tsp. cumin
- 1 tsp. sea salt

Directions:

1. Pour coconut oil into a large skillet. Place on the stove over medium heat for about 1 minute.
2. Add the garlic and onions and cook for three minutes.
3. Add the mushrooms and crumbled tofu. Cook for 10 minutes, stirring occasionally. If the tofu starts to stick, add 1 tbsp. water to the skillet.
4. Add turmeric, cumin, salt, nutritional yeast, and spinach. Stir and cook for another three minutes, then serve.

Spicy Egg and Tomato Sauce Skillet

Servings: 4

Prep and cook time: 15 minutes

Ingredients:

- 2 tbsp. olive oil
- 4 eggs
- ½ cup onions (chopped)
- 2 garlic cloves (minced)
- ½ corn kernels
- 1 cup kale (chopped)
- 1 cup tomatoes (chopped)
- ½ tsp. sumac*
- ½ tsp. ras el hanout*
- Sea salt
- Black pepper

*If you can't find the spices sumac or ras el hanout in your local store, you can substitute the same amount of lemon zest or juice for the sumac. For the ras el hanout, you can add ¼ tsp. cumin, an ⅛ tsp. of each: ground ginger, paprika, coriander, cinnamon, all spice, and cloves.

Directions:

1. Place a large skillet on your stove over medium heat; add the oil. Allow the oil to heat for about 1 minute, then add the onions and garlic. Sauté for 3 minutes.
2. Add the corn and kale to the pan. Cook for 2 minutes or until the kale begins to wilt.
3. Add the tomato. Cook for another 2 minutes.
4. Stir in the sumac and ras el hanout (or substitute ingredients).
5. Create four wells in the vegetables and crack the eggs in the wells. Reduce the heat to low, cover, and cook for 5 minutes or until the egg whites have set.
6. Sprinkle it with sea salt and pepper. Serve immediately.

Egg Salad Lettuce Wraps

Servings: 2 wraps

Prep and cook time: 10 minutes

Ingredients:

- 1 tbsp. extra-virgin olive oil
- 6 boiled eggs (peeled and chopped)
- 4 to 6 bibb lettuce leaves
- ¾ cup grape tomatoes (chopped)
- 2 tbsp. red onion (chopped)
- 2 tbsp. basil (fresh, chopped)
- 2 tbsp. white wine vinegar
- ¼ tsp. sea salt

Directions:

1. In a small mixing bowl, whisk the olive oil, vinegar, and salt together, then set aside.
2. In a larger mixing bowl, toss the chopped boiled eggs, tomatoes, onion, and basil.
3. Pour the olive oil mixture over the boiled egg mixture and stir.
4. Layer two to three lettuce leaves on top of each other and scoop ¼ cup of the egg mixture into each leaf. Roll and enjoy.

Shrimp Lettuce Wraps

Servings: 4 wraps

Prep and cook time: 15 minutes

Ingredients:

- 1 tbsp. extra-virgin olive oil
- 1 pound shrimp (cooked, peeled, and deveined)

- 1 carrot (peeled, shredded)
- 1 yellow bell pepper (chopped fine)
- ½ cup cooked black beans (if using canned, drain and rinse)
- ¼ cup cilantro leaves
- 2 limes (¼ cup juice and 1 tbsp. rind)
- ½ tsp. cumin
- ¼ tsp. sea salt
- 4 to 8 large butter lettuce leaves

Directions:

1. Place all ingredients, except the lettuce leaves, into a large bowl and mix thoroughly.
2. Refrigerate for at least 10 minutes, or cover and keep refrigerated until ready to serve.
3. Take a large lettuce leaf and spoon about ⅓ cup of the shrimp mixture in the center. If the leaves are small, you may want to stack two together.
4. Fold the leaves and enjoy!

Sesame Chicken Shredded Veggie Salad

Servings: 2

Prep and cook time: 15 minutes

Ingredients:
- 8 oz. chicken breast
- 1 egg white
- 2 tbsp. sesame seeds
- 2 cups cabbage (shredded)
- 2 carrots (shredded)
- 4 radishes (sliced thin)
- 2 tbsp. tahini

- 2 tsp. liquid aminos or soy sauce
- 2 tsp. rice vinegar
- 1 tsp. honey
- 2 tsp. ginger (fresh, grated)

Directions:

1. Preheat oven to 400°F.
2. Line a baking sheet with parchment paper and set aside.
3. Whisk egg white with 1 tbsp. water and set aside.
4. Place the sesame seeds in a small bowl next to the egg white.
5. Cut your chicken breast into six slices. Dip each slice in the egg white and then the sesame seed. Place the breasts on your baking sheet.
6. Bake the chicken for 10 minutes.
7. As the chicken bakes, prepare your salad. Toss all remaining ingredients into a large salad bowl and set in the refrigerator until ready to serve.
8. Once chicken is baked, place about 1 ½ cup salad on a large plate and top it with three slices of chicken.

Chicken Mango Bowls

Servings: 4

Prep and cook time: 10 minutes

Ingredients:

- 2 tsp. olive oil
- 1 cup organic chicken broth
- 2 cups cooked brown rice
- 4 chicken breasts (boneless, skinless)
- 2 mangos (peeled, diced)
- 1 bell pepper (chopped)
- 2 green onions (chopped)

- 1 garlic clove (minced)
- 2 tbsp. fresh mint (chopped)
- 1 tbsp. lime juice
- 1 tsp. lime zest
- ¼ tsp. sea salt
- ¼ tsp. black pepper

Directions:

1. Pour oil into a large skillet. Place on the stove over medium-high heat.
2. Season the chicken with salt and pepper, then set in the skillet. Reduce heat to medium; cook the chicken for 2 minutes on each side.
3. Add the mangos, bell pepper, onions, mint, lime juice, zest, and garlic into the skillet. Pour in the broth. Cover partially and cook for 5 minutes or until the chicken is cooked all the way through.
4. Add the rice, stir, and cook for 1 minute.
5. Divide into four equal servings—1 chicken breast and 1 cup rice mixture per serving—and enjoy.

Chicken-Zucchini Noodle Bowl

Servings: 4

Prep and cook time: 10 minutes

Ingredients:

- 1 tbsp. extra-virgin olive oil
- 3 cups chicken breast (cooked, cubed)
- 1 tbsp. lemon juice
- 1 tsp. wasabi paste
- 1 tbsp. honey
- ½ cup Greek yogurt

- 4 cups baby spinach
- 2 zucchini (use a spiralizer to make into noodles)
- 16 grape tomatoes (cut in half)
- 1 avocado (pit removed, sliced)
- ½ tsp. sea salt

Directions:

1. In a small mixing bowl, whisk together the oil, lemon juice, wasabi, honey, yogurt, and salt for the dressing. Set in the refrigerator.
2. Take four bowls and divide the spinach, zucchini noodles, grape tomatoes, and avocado evenly.
3. Add about ¼ cup cooked chicken breast to each bowl.
4. Top with two tablespoons of the dressing and enjoy!

Salmon and Edamummus Toast

Servings: 4

Prep and cook time: 5 minutes

Ingredients:

- 1 tbsp. extra-virgin olive oil
- 3 tbsp. water
- 4 oz. cold smoked salmon (sliced thin)
- 1 ⅔ cup of edamame (frozen, defrosted, shelled)
- 1 ½ tsp. tahini
- 1 ½ tbsp. lemon juice
- 1 tsp. lemon zest
- 1 garlic clove
- 1 cucumber (sliced into thin ribbons)
- 1 cup baby salad greens
- 4 pieces of whole-grain or rye bread

Directions:

1. Place your bread into the toaster to toast.
2. Combine the edamame, tahini, lemon juice and zest, garlic, and olive oil. Begin to process, add 1 tbsp. water in at a time until you have a smooth thick mixture.
3. Toast bread and spread two generous tablespoons of the edamame mixture over the toast.
4. Top with salmon, cucumber ribbons, and baby greens. Enjoy!

IF Recipes

Berry Crisp

Servings: 6

Prep and cook time: 45 minutes

Ingredients:

- 2 cups cherries (seeds removed, cut in half)
- 2 cups blueberries
- 1 tsp. cinnamon
- 1 tsp. nutmeg
- ¼ cup almond milk
- 1 tsp. pure vanilla extract
- 1 tsp. pure almond extract
- 1 tsp. agar-agar, arrowroot, or xanthan gum
- ½ tbsp. cornstarch
- 1 ½ cup old-fashioned oats
- ¼ cup brown sugar
- 2 tbsp. honey
- 1 cup Greek yogurt

Directions:

1. Preheat oven to 350°F.
2. Spray an 8x8 baking pan with cooking spray and set aside.
3. In a medium mixing bowl, combine the cherries, blueberries, cinnamon, nutmeg, almond milk, vanilla, agar-agar, cornstarch, and honey. Stir together thoroughly, then transfer to the baking pan.
4. In a small mixing bowl, combine the oats, brown sugar, and Greek yogurt. Spread over the berry mixture.
5. Place in the oven and bake for 45 minutes.
6. Allow to cool slightly before serving.

Berry Peach Smoothie Bowl

Servings: 2 bowls

Prep and cook time: 5 minutes

Ingredients:

- 1 cup peaches (frozen)
- ¼ cup blueberries
- ¼ cup strawberries
- ¼ cup coconut milk
- ½ cup Greek yogurt
- ½ tsp. pure almond extract
- 1 tsp. chia seeds
- 2 tbsp. almonds
- 1 tbsp. honey

Directions:

1. Add the frozen peaches, coconut milk, yogurt, and almond extract to a blender.
2. Blend until smooth; transfer to a bowl.

3. Top with blueberries, strawberries, chia seeds, almonds, and drizzle with honey.

Avocado Quesadillas

Servings: 2

Prep and cook time: 20 minutes

Ingredients:

- ½ tsp. olive oil
- 1 tomato (chopped)
- 1 avocado (pitted, peeled, chopped)
- 1 tbsp. red onion (chopped)
- 2 tsp. lemon juice
- 4 x 24-inch whole wheat tortillas
- 3 tbsp. fresh coriander (chopped)
- 1 cup sour cream or plain Greek yogurt
- 1 cup Monterey jack cheese (shredded)
- ¼ tsp. sea salt
- ¼ tsp. black pepper
- Hot sauce (optional)

Directions:

1. Mix the tomatoes, avocado, onion, lemon juice, sea salt, black pepper, and ¼ teaspoon hot sauce if you're adding hot sauce. Toss and set to the side.
2. In another mixing bowl, combine the sour cream and coriander, then set aside.
3. Take two of the tortillas and brush one side with olive oil.
4. Set the tortillas broiler with the oil side facing up. Broil for 1 minute.
5. Sprinkle the Monterey jack cheese over the tortilla and broil again until the cheese melts.

6. Spread the avocado and tomato mixture over the tortilla. Place the other tortilla on top, and broil for 1 minute.
7. Carefully remove the quesadillas and cut into four wedges.
8. Top each piece with a little of the sour cream mixture and enjoy.

Cheesy Chicken Salad

Servings: 2

Prep and cook time: 40 minutes (30 minutes chill time)

Ingredients:
- 1 cup chicken breast (cooked, boneless, skinless, cut into cubes)
- 1 celery stick (chopped fine)
- 1 small carrot (shredded)
- ½ cup spinach (chopped)
- ¼ tsp. parsley
- 1 tbsp. mayonnaise
- 2 tbsp. sour cream
- ¼ cup sharp cheddar cheese (shredded)
- 2 tsp. Dijon mustard

Directions:
1. Place everything into a large mixing bowl and mix thoroughly.
2. Cover and chill in the refrigerator for at least 30 minutes, then enjoy!

Cobb Salad

Servings: 2

Prep and cook time: 15 minutes

Ingredients:

- 3 hard-boiled eggs
- ½ lb. roasted turkey breast (chopped)
- ½ head of lettuce (chopped)
- ½ bunch watercress
- 1 bunch chicory lettuce
- ½ head of romaine lettuce (chopped)
- 1 tomato (chopped)
- 1 avocado (pitted, peeled, chopped)
- 1 tbsp. chives (chopped)
- ½ cup blue cheese crumbles

For dressing:

- 2 tbsp. extra virgin olive oil
- 2 garlic cloves (minced)
- 2 tbsp. water
- ½ tsp. Worcestershire sauce
- 2 tbsp. balsamic or red wine vinegar
- 1 tbsp. lemon juice
- **⅛ tsp. Dijon mustard**
- ½ tbsp. honey
- ¾ tsp. sea salt
- ½ tsp. black pepper

Directions:

1. In a food processor, combine all the dressing ingredients except the olive oil.
2. Process until you have a smooth mixture, then slowly add in olive oil. Process until thoroughly combined. Set it in the refrigerator.
3. On a large long serving plate, arrange the lettuce into rows.
4. Layer the remaining ingredients in rows above the lettuce. Set in the refrigerator until ready to serve.

5. Drizzle the dressing over the salad when serving.

Mediterranean Salad with Quinoa and Millet

Servings: 4

Prep and cook time: 40 minutes

Ingredients:

- 1 tbsp. olive oil
- ½ cup millet
- ½ cup quinoa
- 1 ¾ cups water (divided)
- 1 English cucumber (diced)
- 1 tomato (seeds removed, diced)
- 1 sweet pepper (seeds removed, diced)
- ½ red onion (diced)
- 1 garlic clove (minced)
- 10 oz. can white beans (drained)
- ¼ tsp. cayenne pepper
- 1 tsp. dill
- ¼ cup feta cheese (crumbled)
- ¼ cup pine nuts
- 1 lemon (juice and zest)
- ½ tsp. sea salt
- ½ tsp. black pepper

Directions:

1. In a saucepan, add 1 cup water. Turn the heat to high and bring it to a boil. Then add the millet and boil for 5 minutes. Turn off the heat, cover, and allow the millet to sit for 10 minutes.
2. In another saucepan, add ¾ cup water. Turn the heat to high and bring it to a boil. Then add the quinoa, reduce heat to medium-low, cover, and for 15 minutes.

3. Add all ingredients into a large mixing bowl. Mix thoroughly and serve.

Cauli-Popcorn

Servings: 4

Prep and cook time: 1 hour 10 minutes

Ingredients:

- 4 tbsp. olive oil
- 1 cauliflower head (trimmed, cored, cut to bite-size florets)
- 1 tsp. sea salt

Directions:

1. Preheat oven to 425°F.
2. Toss the cauliflower florets in a large mixing bowl with the oil and salt.
3. Spread the cauliflower over a baking sheet lined with parchment paper. Bake for 1 hour or until the cauliflower is a nice golden brown. Toss four times.
4. Remove from the oven and enjoy!

Shredded Brussel Sprouts

Servings: 6

Prep and cook time: 30 minutes

Ingredients:

- 2 slices of bacon
- 1 lb. brussels sprouts (trimmed, sliced thin)
- 1 yellow onion (sliced thin)

- 1 tsp. Dijon mustard
- 1 tbsp. apple cider vinegar
- ¾ cup water
- ¼ tsp. sea salt

Directions:

1. Cook the bacon in a large skillet about 7 minutes over medium heat. Remove from the skillet and set on paper towels.
2. In the same skillet, add the sliced onions and cook for 3 minutes. Stir occasionally.
3. Pour the water into the skillet, then add the Dijon mustard and sliced Brussel sprouts. Stir occasionally and cook for 6 minutes.
4. Add the vinegar to the skillet and stir.
5. Remove from the heat.
6. Crumble bacon on top, sprinkle with the salt, then serve.

Roasted Broccoli

Servings: 4

Prep and cook time: 15 minutes

Ingredients:

- 2 tbsp. olive oil
- 1 lb. broccoli florets
- 1 garlic clove (minced)
- 2 tbsp. unsalted butter
- ½ tsp. lemon zest
- 2 tbsp. lemon juice
- 2 tbsp. toasted pine nuts
- ½ tsp. sea salt
- ½ tsp. black pepper

Directions:

1. Preheat oven to 475°F.
2. In a large mixing bowl, toss the broccoli florets with olive oil, sea salt, and black pepper.
3. Spread the broccoli over a baking sheet and place in the oven.
4. Roast for 6 minutes, toss, then roast for another 6 minutes.
5. As the broccoli is roasting, melt butter in a sauce pan on the stove over medium heat.
6. Once the butter has melted, add garlic and lemon zest. Stir continuously for 1 minute.
7. Remove from heat, then stir in the lemon juice.
8. Once the broccoli is done, transfer it to a serving plate.
9. Drizzle the butter-lemon mixture over top and top with pine nuts before serving.

Black Bean Soup

Servings: 4

Prep and cook time:

Ingredients:

- 1 tbsp. olive oil
- 1 yellow onion (chopped)
- 1 small red onion (chopped fine)
- 3 garlic cloves (minced)
- 2 x 14.5 oz. cans of black beans (drain and rinsed)
- 2 cups chicken broth
- 1 tbsp. cumin
- ¼ cup cilantro (fresh, chopped fine)
- ½ tsp. sea salt
- ½ tsp. black pepper

Directions:

1. Place a medium saucepan on the stove with the oil in it, turn the heat to medium. Allow the oil to heat for 1 minute.
2. Add the yellow onion to the pan and sauté for 5 minutes.
3. Add the garlic and cook for 2 minutes.
4. Add one can of the black beans and the chicken broth. Simmer for 5 minutes.
5. Remove the pan from the heat and use an immersion blender to blend everything together. If you do not have an immersion blender, you can use a stand-alone blender, but you may have to work in batches.
6. Set the saucepan back over medium heat. Add the other can of black beans, cumin, salt, pepper, and red onion. Allow everything to simmer for 10 minutes.
7. Serve with fresh cilantro overtop.

Sweet Potato Curry with Chickpeas and Spinach

Servings: 6

Prep and cook time: 45 minutes

Ingredients:
- 4 tsp. olive oil (divided)
- ½ tsp. salt
- ½ tsp. black pepper
- 1 large sweet onion (sliced thin)
- 2 cups spinach (stems removed, chopped)
- 2 sweet potatoes (peeled, diced)
- 2 cups tomatoes (dice)
- 2 tbsp. curry powder
- 1 tbsp. cumin
- 1 tsp. cinnamon
- 14.5 oz. can of chickpeas (drained, rinsed)

- ½ cup water
- 1 ½ cups cooked brown rice

Directions:

1. **Preheat oven to 450°F.**
2. Toss the diced sweet potato in a bowl with 2 tsp. olive oil, salt, and black pepper.
3. Spread the potatoes over a baking sheet and place in the oven and back for 30 minutes. Toss after 15 minutes.
4. While the potatoes roast, place a large skillet on the stove with the remaining 2 tsp. oil. Heat over medium heat.
5. Add the onions and sauté for 3 minutes.
6. Add the curry powder, cumin, and cinnamon. Stir to coat the onions.
7. Add the tomatoes, chickpeas, and water. Raise the heat to medium-high and allow the liquids to reach a simmer.
8. Add the spinach. You may want to do a handful at a time so there is enough room in the skillet. Stir, cover, lower the heat to medium, and simmer for 5 minutes.
9. Once the potatoes finish roasting, add them to the skillet. Stir and simmer for another 5 minutes.
10. Serve your sweet potato mixture over ¼ cup brown rice.

Mediterranean Chicken with Avocado Tapenade

Servings: 4

Prep and cook time:

Ingredients:
- 3 tbsp. olive oil (divided)
- 4 chicken breasts (boneless, skinless, halved)
- 3 garlic cloves (1 minced, 2 roasted and mashed)
- 1 tomato (chopped)

- ¼ cup pimento-stuffed olives (sliced thin)
- 1 avocado (pitted, chopped)
- 3 tbsp. capers
- 2 tbsp. basil leaves (sliced thin)
- 2 lemons (1 tbsp. of zest, 4 tbsp. juice divided)
- ½ tsp. sea salt
- ½ tsp. black pepper

Directions:

1. Place the chicken breast in a sealable bag with the lemon zest, 2 tbsp. lemon juice, 2 tbsp. olive oil, minced garlic, salt, and pepper. Place in the refrigerator for at least 30 minutes.
2. In a large mixing bowl, toss the tomatoes, olives, and avocados. Set aside.
3. Whisk together 2 tbsp. lemon juice, roasted garlic, and ½ tsp. olive oil. Pour over the tomato mixture and toss. Set in the refrigerator until ready to serve.
4. Set a grill pan on your stove and heat over medium heat.
5. Once heated, place your marinated chicken breast on the grill. Cook for 5 minutes on each side or until completely done.
6. Serve cooked chicken topped with chilled avocado tapenade.

Sheet Pan Chicken and Vegetables

Servings: 4

Prep and cook time: 40 minutes

Ingredients:

- 3 tbsp. olive oil (divided)
- 4 chicken thighs (skin on)
- 1 ½ cups Brussel sprouts (halved)
- 4 carrots (cut to thick sticks)
- 1 tsp. herbes de provence

Directions:

1. Preheat oven to 400
2. In a large mixing bowl, add the Brussel sprouts, carrots, and 1 ½ teaspoons olive oil. Sprinkle ½ tsp. herbes de provence on top and rub to ensure all the vegetables are nicely coated. Transfer to a large sheet pan.
3. Place chicken thigh, one at a time, in the same bowl, with 1 ½ tbsp. olive oil and ½ tsp. herbes de provence. Sprinkle with salt and pepper. Use your hands to rub the herbs into the chicken. Transfer the chicken to the sheet pan.
4. Place the pan in the oven and bake for 35 minutes or until the chicken is cooked all the way through.
5. Remove the pan from the oven and serve.

Grilled Salmon with Lemon

Servings: 4

Prep and cook time: 1 hour, 20 minutes

Ingredients:

- 3 tbsp. olive oil
- 1 ½ lbs. salmon filets
- 4 tbsp. green onions (chopped fine)
- 1 onion (sliced in rings)
- 1 lemon (sliced thin)
- 3 tbsp. liquid aminos or soy sauce
- 4 tbsp. honey
- 2 tsp. dill
- 1 tsp. garlic powder
- ½ tsp. sea salt
- ½ tsp. black pepper

Directions:

1. In a small mixing bowl, whisk together the olive oil, honey, liquid aminos, and green onions. Set aside.
2. Take salmon filets and sprinkle them with the dill, garlic powder, sea salt, and black pepper. Set the filets in a shallow dish, then pour the oil mixture over the salmon. Cover and chill for 1 hour in the refrigerator.
3. Heat a grill pan or outdoor grill.
4. Place the salmon filets on the grill and discard the marinade. Place the sliced onions and lemons over the salmon.
5. Cover and cook for 15 minutes over medium heat or until the salmon is cooked thoroughly.
6. Serve with your favorite grilled vegetables, over salad, or with brown rice and vegetables.

Vegan Tacos with Pickled Onions

Servings: 8

Prep and cook time: 45 minutes

Ingredients:

- 2 tbsp. olive oil
- 14 oz. silken tofu (pat dry, cut into 10-inch cubes)
- 1 tsp. smoked paprika
- ½ tsp. cayenne pepper
- 1 tsp. ground cumin
- ¼ head of cabbage (shredded)
- 1 avocado (chopped)
- 1 red onion (sliced fine)
- ¼ cup apple cider vinegar
- 1 tbsp. sugar
- 1 ½ tsp. fine sea salt (divided)
- 8 small whole wheat tortillas

Directions:

1. Pour the vinegar into a small saucepan. Place over medium heat.
2. Add the sugar and 1 tsp. salt. Stir occasionally for 5 minutes.
3. Place the onions into a jar or bowl and pour the hot vinegar on top. Let the onions sit for at least 30 minutes.
4. Place a large skillet on your stove and add the olive oil. Turn the heat to medium.
5. Add the paprika, cayenne, and cumin to the skillet. All the spices cook for only 1 minute. Carefully add the tofu in a single layer. You may need to work in batches.
6. Cook the tofu on each side for 2 minutes or until golden brown.
7. Once the tofu is cooked, build your tacos. Take a tortilla and add a few pieces of tofu. Top with shredded lettuce, avocado, and pickled onions.

Conclusion

Turning 50 should be celebrated. It's a major event that you shouldn't fear or dread. While many women over 50 struggle with their weight, health, and confidence, you don't have to. You can take control of your health at any age!

Just because you're getting older doesn't mean you have to settle for all the ailments that come with aging. You can adopt healthy habits and make long-term lifestyle changes that will make you feel 20 years younger. Throughout this book, you've learned the best ways to approach your health, whether in your 40s, 50s or older. This information is designed with menopausal and post-menopausal women in mind because of the significant changes your body is going through that make weight loss and optimal health a struggle.

Transitioning to a nutritious diet, whether whole food or a plant-based approach like the Mediterranean diet, is the first step to the vibrant life you seek. You've learned how to reduce the risk of many health conditions by being more aware and mindful of what you consume. You can boost the health benefits of a nutritious diet by finding a suitable fasting method that is comfortable for you. Whether you fast for 14 hours or 18, you know that letting your body shift into fat-burning mode is an effective way to lose weight and sync your body to its natural rhythms.

Don't let getting older keep you from being physically active, either. Moving your body will keep your bones strong and ensure you have the muscle mass to keep you going for another 20 or more years. You don't have to spend hours at the gym or push yourself to exhaustion. Simple movements, like yoga and walking, can keep you fit.

You now have the information you need to maintain a healthy mind and body. Remember that boosting your immune system entails a holistic multi-step approach. You can eat healthy foods and still quickly tire if you don't exercise. You can exercise and still have a weak immune system if you lack sleep. Creating healthy habits helps you get stronger, but not doing the other necessary things can counteract your progress and weaken your defense system. When you reach your golden years, make it worthwhile by choosing to be healthy and strong to enjoy your life ahead with vitality and stamina. Being 50 and over is just a number. Choose to be your best version by taking care of and loving yourself.

I hope that you feel more confident about your golden years. I hope you don't dread another birthday and that you take the first steps to feel healthier, happy, and vibrant. I hope you share with other women what has resonated most with you on these pages and what works best for you. You can encourage and support other women to take control of their health by leaving a review. Share the benefits you experience by practicing what you learned throughout this book.

Thank you for allowing me to share your healthy lifestyle journey, and I wish you many more years of health, energy, and joy!

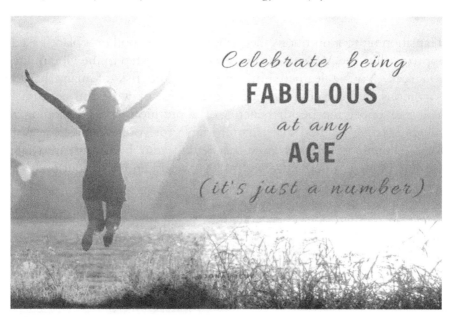

References

A quote by Hippocrates. (n.d.). Good Reads. https://www.goodreads.com/quotes/62262-let-food-be-thy-medicine-and-medicine-be-thy-food

Agarwal, N. (2020, May 2). *Food synergy: Know the foods which must be eaten together.* NDTV.com. https://www.ndtv.com/health/food-synergy-know-the-foods-which-must-be-eaten-together-2221920

Al Bander, Z., Nitert, M.D., Mousa, A., & Naderpoor, N. (2020). The Gut Microbiota and Inflammation: An Overview. *International Journal of Environmental Research and Public Health, 17*(20). https://doi.org/10.3390/ijerph17207618

Aleknavičius, K. (2021, November 22). *13 surprising benefits of intermittent fasting that every faster should know about.* Do Fasting. https://blog.dofasting.com/intermittent-fasting-benefits/

Alexis, A. C. (2022, May 27). *Intermittent fasting: Is it all it's cracked up to be?* Medical News Today. https://www.medicalnewstoday.com/articles/intermittent-fasting-is-it-all-its-cracked-up-to-be#Benefits

American Heart Association Editorial Staff. (2016, October 31). *What is high blood pressure?* Www.heart.org. https://www.heart.org/en/health-topics/high-blood-pressure/the-facts-about-high-blood-pressure/what-is-high-blood-pressure

Bates, A. (2018, August 6). *3 ways intermittent fasting can balance your hormones.* Autumn Elle Nutrition. https://www.autumnellenutrition.com/post/3-ways-intermittent-fasting-can-balance-your-hormones

Berman, R. (2021, April 22). *Gut bacteria and inflammation: The role of diet.* Medical News Today. https://www.medicalnewstoday.com/articles/how-diet-influences-gut-bacteria-and-inflammation#Eating-a-gut-healthier-diet

Brighten, Dr. J. (2022, January 14). *Intermittent fasting for women.* Dr. Jolene Brighten. https://drbrighten.com/intermittent-fasting-womens-health/

Brill, J. B. (n.d.). *Intermittent fasting and the Mediterranean diet—A match made in health heaven.* ModifyHealth. https://modifyhealth.com/blogs/blog/intermittent-fasting-and-the-mediterranean-diet-a-match-made-in-health-heaven

Brown, L. (n.d.). *Interesting facts about glucose.* LIVESTRONG. https://www.livestrong.com/article/229319-interesting-glucose-facts/

Brubaker, M. (2017, January 12). *Exercise … it does a body good: 20 minutes can act as anti-inflammatory.* UC San Diego. https://health.ucsd.edu/news/releases/pages/2017-01-12-exercise-can-act-as-anti-inflammatory.aspx#:~:text=%E2%80%9COur%20study%20shows%0a%20workout

Brummert, D. (2021, April 26). *Gut health: Why it matters.* Orlando Health. https://www.orlandohealth.com/content-hub/gut-health-why-it-matters

Byrne, C. (2021, August 11). *What's the difference between blood sugar and A1C?* Silver Sneakers. https://www.silversneakers.com/blog/whats-the-difference-between-blood-sugar-and-a1c/

Caporuscio, J. (2019, March 30). *What are the most healthful oils?* Medical News Today. https://www.medicalnewstoday.com/articles/324844

Charleson, K. (2022, April 26). *Why it's important to monitor glucose levels.* Very Well Health. https://www.verywellhealth.com/glucose-levels-what-you-should-know-5116621

Cleveland Clinic. (2021, July 28). *Inflammation: What is it, causes, symptoms & treatment.* https://my.clevelandclinic.org/health/symptoms/21660-inflammation

Cleveland Clinic. (2022, March 3). *Intermittent fasting: 4 different types explained.* Health Essentials from Cleveland Clinic. https://health.clevelandclinic.org/intermittent-fasting-4-different-types-explained/

Cleveland Clinic. (2019, November 13). *Hyperosmolar hyperglycemic syndrome.* Cleveland Clinic. https://my.clevelandclinic.org/health/diseases/21147-hyperosmolar-hyperglycemic-syndrome#:~:text=What%20is%20hyperosmolar%20hyperglycemic%20syndrome

Coconut Oil. (n.d.). Harvard T.H. Chan School of Public Health. https://www.hsph.harvard.edu/nutritionsource/food-features/coconut-oil/#:~:text=Coconut%20oil%20is%20made%20by

Davids Landau, M. (2020, March 17). *10 surprising facts about female hormones that every woman should know.* Prevention. https://www.prevention.com/health/a31672318/female-hormones/

Davis, C. P. (2021, March 22). *How long do you need to fast for autophagy?* MedicineNet. https://www.medicinenet.com/how_long_do_you_need_to_fast_for_autophagy/article.htm#:~:text=Intermittent%20fasting%20is%20a%20possible

Dietary fats, oils and cholesterol. (n.d.). Heart and Stroke Foundation of Canada. https://www.heartandstroke.ca/healthy-living/healthy-eating/fats-and-oils

Difference Between Fat And Cholesterol. (n.d.). BYJUS. https://byjus.com/chemistry/difference-between-fat-and-cholesterol/

Different cooking oils and their health benefits. (2021, April 6). Integris Health. https://integrisok.com/resources/on-your-health/2021/april/different-cooking-oils-and-their-health-benefits

Elflein, J. (2022, May 7). *Top 10 causes of death among women U.S. 2019.* Statista. https://www.statista.com/statistics/233289/distribution-of-the-10-leading-causes-of-death-among-women/

Erlich, E. (n.d.). *What women over 50 should know about intermittent fasting.* Nutritious Life. https://nutritiouslife.com/eat-empowered/intermittent-fasting-women-over-50/

Geurin, L. (2021, December 23). *42 intermittent fasting quotes to motivate you.* Lori Geurin Wellness for Life. https://lorigeurin.com/intermittent-fasting-quotes/

Glossary. (n.d.). Nutrition Authority. https://nutritionauthority.com/glossary/

Grace & Silas. (n.d.). *8 intermittent fasting hacks that'll make your life easier.* Chasing Foxes. https://www.chasingfoxes.com/8-intermittent-fasting-hacks-thatll-making-your-life-easier/

Grey, H. (2019, October 22). *The Mediterranean diet can help keep your gut happy.* Healthline. https://www.healthline.com/health-news/heres-what-to-eat-to-keep-your-gut-happy#Mediterranean-diet-might-reduce-inflammation

Gupta, L. (2016, August 22). *Different types of cooking oils and their benefits.* Health Kart. https://www.healthkart.com/connect/different-types-of-cooking-oils-and-their-benefits/bid-4975

Gunnars, K. (2021, May 13). *10 health benefits of intermittent fasting.* Healthline. https://www.healthline.com/nutrition/10-health-benefits-of-intermittent-fasting#The-bottom-line

Gupta, S. (2020, November 26). *Struggling with hormonal imbalance? Cut these 6 foods out of your diet.* Health Shots. https://www.healthshots.com/healthy-eating/nutrition/struggling-with-hormonal-imbalance-cut-these-6-foods-out-of-your-diet/

Harvard Health Publishing. (2020, May 1). *Mediterranean diet linked to lower inflammation, healthy aging.* Harvard Health. https://www.health.harvard.edu/staying-healthy/mediterranean-diet-linked-to-lower-inflammation-healthy-aging

Harvard Health Publishing. (2021, December 16). *Foods that fight inflammation.* Harvard Health; Harvard Health. https://www.health.harvard.edu/staying-healthy/foods-that-fight-inflammation

Heart UK. (n.d.). *What is cholesterol?* https://www.heartuk.org.uk/cholesterol/what-is-cholesterol

Intermittent fasting and hormone balance. (n.d.). . https://www.mealprep.com.au/intermittent-fasting/intermittent-fasting-and-hormone-balance/

Intermittent fasting: 4 different types explained. (n.d.). Health Essentials from Cleveland Clinic. https://health.clevelandclinic.org/intermittent-fasting-4-different-types-explained/

Iwasa, T., Matsuzaki, T., Yano, K., & Irahara, M. (2017). Gonadotropin-Inhibitory Hormone Plays Roles in Stress-Induced Reproductive Dysfunction. *Front. Endocrinol, 8,* 62. https://doi.org/https://doi.org/10.3389/fendo.2017.00062

Jackson, C. (2022, January 27). *Researchers uncover link between gut microbiome and inflammatory diseases.* GEN—Genetic Engineering and Biotechnology News. https://www.genengnews.com/news/researchers-uncover-link-between-gut-microbiome-and-inflammatory-diseases/

John Hopkins Medicine. (n.d.). *Intermittent fasting: What is it, and how does it work?* Johns Hopkins Medicine. https://www.hopkinsmedicine.org/health/wellness-and-prevention/intermittent-fasting-what-is-it-and-how-does-it-work

Kandola, A. (2018, November 7). *Top 5 intermittent fasting benefits ranked.* Medical News Today. https://www.medicalnewstoday.com/articles/323605#takeaway

Krans, B. (2020, June 29). *Balanced diet: What is it and how to achieve it.* Healthline. https://www.healthline.com/health/balanced-diet#putting-it-together

Kresser, C. (2019, February 19). *How industrial seed oils are making us sick.* Chris Kresser. https://chriskresser.com/how-industrial-seed-oils-are-making-us-sick/

Kumar, D. (2020, April 17). *9 essential oils you should add to your skin and hair care regime.* Swirlster. https://swirlster.ndtv.com/beauty/essential-oils-for-beautiful-skin-and-hair-benefits-and-how-to-use-2213449

Landsverk, G. (2021, November 4). *Eating protein 4 times a day combined with fasting may help you burn belly fat faster than calorie cutting alone, research suggests.* Insider. https://www.insider.com/eating-high-protein-while-intermittent-fasting-may-help-weight-loss-2021-11

LDL and HDL cholesterol: "Bad" and "good" cholesterol. (2020, January 31). Centers for Disease Control and Prevention. https://www.cdc.gov/cholesterol/ldl_hdl.htm

Lin, S., Oliveira, M.L., Gabel, K., Kalam, F., Cienfuegos, S., Ezpeleta, M., Bhutani, S., & Varady, K. A. (2021). *Does the weight loss efficacy of alternate day fasting differ according to sex and menopausal status?* Nutrition, Metabolism and Cardiovascular Diseases, 31(2), 641–649. https://doi.org/10.1016/j.numecd.2020.10.018

Martin, M. (2021, November 7). *Chair squats*. Melio Guide: The Guide to a Stronger You. https://melioguide.com/osteoporosis-exercises/chair-squats/

Mayo Clinic Staff. (2020, February 23). *Trans fat: Double trouble for your heart*. https://www.mayoclinic.org/diseases-conditions/high-blood-cholesterol/in-depth/trans-fat/art-20046114

Mayo Clinic Staff. (2021, March 12). *Menopause weight gain: Stop the middle age spread*. Mayo Clinic. https://www.mayoclinic.org/healthy-lifestyle/womens-health/in-depth/menopause-weight-gain/art-20046058

Mayo Clinic Staff. (2022, September 3). *Triglycerides: Why do they matter?* Mayo Clinic. https://www.mayoclinic.org/diseases-conditions/high-blood-cholesterol/in-depth/triglycerides/art-20048186

Mediterranean diet linked to lower inflammation, healthy aging. (2020, May 1). Harvard Health. https://www.health.harvard.edu/staying-healthy/mediterranean-diet-linked-to-lower-inflammation-healthy-aging

Merschel, M. (2021, April 1). *AHA News: Why you should pay attention to inflammation*. Health Day. https://consumer.healthday.com/aha-news-why-you-should-pay-attention-to-inflammation-2651317804.html

Migala, J. (2022, February 7). *Whole-foods diet 101: A complete beginner's guide*. Everyday Health. https://www.everydayhealth.com/diet-nutrition/whole-foods-diet/

Migala, J., & Lawler, M. (2022, June 6). *A complete Mediterranean diet food list and 14-day meal plan*. Everyday Health. https://www.everydayhealth.com/mediterranean-diet/complete-mediterranean-diet-food-list-day-meal-plan/

Moore, C. (2019, March 4). *Positive daily affirmations: Is there science behind it?* Positive Psychology. https://positivepsychology.com/daily-affirmations/

More Key Topics. (n.d.). My Plate. https://www.myplate.gov/eat-healthy/more-key-topics

Morgan, M. (2022, July 26). *Intermittent fasting for women over 50 2022: What you should know.* Healthcanal.com. https://www.healthcanal.com/life-style-fitness/intermittent-fasting-women-over-50

My Fitness Pal's Recipes. (2020, March 18). *11 20-minute recipes with up to 32 grams of protein.* My Fitness Pal Blog. https://blog.myfitnesspal.com/11-20-minute-recipes-under-355-calories/

Nazario, B. (2020, August 19). *Over 50? These problems can sneak up on you.* WebMD. https://www.webmd.com/healthy-aging/ss/slideshow-health-problems-after-50

NIA Scientist. (2021, September 30). *Sleep problems and menopause: What can I do?* National Institute on Aging. https://www.nia.nih.gov/health/sleep-problems-and-menopause-what-can-i-do

Our 32 top intermittent fasting recipes. (n.d.). Food. https://www.food.com/ideas/intermittent-fasting-recipes-6939#c-798529

Pacheco, D. (2022, September 12). *Sleep and blood glucose levels.* Sleep Foundation. https://www.sleepfoundation.org/physical-health/sleep-and-blood-glucose-levels#:~:text=A%20study%20of%20people%20with

Satrazemis, E. (2019, June 30). *Clean eating food list: What to eat and what to avoid.* Trifecta. https://www.trifectanutrition.com/blog/clean-eating-food-list-what-to-eat-and-what-to-avoid

Schuchmann, C. (2020, August 26). *Is full-fat food better than low-fat or fat-free food?* UChicagoMedicine. https://www.uchicagomedicine.org/forefront/gastrointestinal-articles/which-are-healthier-low-fat-or-full-fat-foods

Stanton, B. (2022). *Intermittent fasting for women over 50: 7 tips for success.* Carb Manager. https://www.carbmanager.com/article/ygj3xheaaawus2xa/intermittent-fasting-for-women-over-50-7-tips-for/

Stanton, B., & O'Neil, T. (2021). *How to choose an intermittent fasting schedule.* Carb Manager. https://www.carbmanager.com/article/yoherxeaaceazayu/how-to-choose-an-intermittent-fasting-schedule/

Summer, J. (2022, June 24). *Why intermittent fasting can lead to better sleep.* Sleep Foundation. https://www.sleepfoundation.org/physical-health/intermittent-fasting-sleep

The Live Better Team. (n.d.). *You can't have one without the other: How body systems are connected.* Revere Health. https://reverehealth.com/live-better/how-body-systems-connected/

Thorpe, J. (2019, May 4). *20 things no one ever told you about inflammation.* Bustle. https://www.bustle.com/p/20-facts-about-inflammation-no-one-ever-told-you-17040269

Trumpfeller, G. (2020, March 20). *Everything you need to know about autophagy: When, why, and how.* Simple.life Blog. https://simple.life/blog/autophagy/

Tsigalou, C., Konstantinidis, T., Paraschaki, A., Stavropoulou, E., Voidarou, C., & Bezirtzoglou, E. (2020). Mediterranean Diet as a Tool to Combat Inflammation and Chronic Diseases. An Overview. *Biomedicines, 8*(7), 201. https://doi.org/10.3390/biomedicines8070201

Typical intestinal bacteria. (n.d.). Otsuka Pharmaceutical Co., Ltd. https://www.otsuka.co.jp/en/health-and-illness/fiber/for-body/intestinal-flora/

Vetter, C. (2022, February 9). *Intermittent fasting: What can you eat or drink?* Zoe. https://joinzoe.com/learn/what-to-eat-or-drink-while-intermittent-fasting

Vitti, A. (2021, November 2). *Intermittent fasting and hormonal health: What you need to know.* Flo Living. https://www.floliving.com/intermittent-fasting/

What's the connection between gut biomes and inflammation? (n.d.). MDVIP. https://www.mdvip.com/about-mdvip/blog/whats-connection-between-gut-biomes-and-inflammation

Why you need unsaturated fats in your diet. (2022, August 24). Cleveland Clinic. https://health.clevelandclinic.org/the-skinny-on-unsaturated-fats-why-you-need-them-the-best-sources/

Wright, S. A., & Dias, A. (2022, August 18). *Everything you need to know about glucose.* Healthline; Healthline Media. https://www.healthline.com/health/glucose#how-glucose-works

Zelman, K. M. (2020, August 4). *How much do you know about fats and oils?* WebMD. https://www.webmd.com/food-recipes/rm-quiz-fats-and-oils

Image References

Anon, S. (n.d.). *Sport and healthy woman tying her shoes. [Image].* Shutterstock. https://www.shutterstock.com/catalog/collections/2991369965300352990-03f1c578ff646e86861bd1cfa06ca8a05db098d922d6525b50fcc057eb0555b2

By-Studio. (n.d.). *Happy jumping woman. [Image].* Shutterstock. https://www.shutterstock.com/catalog/collections/2991383639167600063-72abd179a4e729785d68cf2eb138b2a73139c3a5d3c05f57a9531bb134cb95ac

Daisy, D. (n.d.). *Full frame shot of foods containing unhealthy or bad carbohydrates.* *[Image].* Shutterstock.https://www.shutterstock.com/catalog/collections/2992558770128684555-cae50f427b04bd949f79075f4469f3ff2cd5cfb9bc4dc82a700337b54dc26ccb

Elenadesign. (n.d.). *Healthy salad bowl with quinoa, tomatoes.* *[Image].* Shutterstock. https://www.shutterstock.com/catalog/collections/2991062864904587002-0adaf8e15f0e728677befebab2e11dc59548f0325bb49a2ed117ecc70507ffb2

Fizkes. (n.d.). *Happy fresh mature middle aged woman.* *[Image].* Shutterstock. https://www.shutterstock.com/catalog/collections/2991339942631704149-566bf9b3715a2efd29a42d7c30e8d92069e4cd1a6f673194e90fa76f1c3c10cc

Marekuliasz. (n.d.). *Respect my hormones - humorous warning.* *[Image].* Shutterstock. https://www.shutterstock.com/catalog/collections/2991362684374484848-a9b2a8e8d4ccc8f4f70f2b66d5eddd71eb5b44be70bf5bfc092e627c624574a4

Marganingsih, M. (n.d.). *Inspirational motivational quote.* *[Image].* Shutterstock. https://www.shutterstock.com/catalog/collections/2992546942191404098-7ee64e48e7146bdadefd632e7cd74eaae2a8a37fcdc4e772489159acfb93420a

McDonald, S. (2020, September 20). *[Granola and fruit parfaits].* *[Image].* Unsplash. https://unsplash.com/photos/XGanQ3jivhg

Monticello. (n.d.). *Composition with variety of organic food.* *[Image].* Shutterstock. https://www.shutterstock.com/catalog/collections/299109224 0123692888- d4e92ad35b89a8945256e7438097f608b7b799168e7cc84999255 5add70bebcf

New Africa. (n.d.). *Different fresh herbs with oils.* *[Image].* Shutterstock. https://www.shutterstock.com/catalog/collections/299107998 2857455051- fe15dfc9a2e2cc8fff1dc110865a52aee6ae821c661c2a726b8412e b0a620220

Nok Lek Travel Lifestyle. (n.d.). *Alarm clock of blue which schedule of meal.* *[Image].* Shutterstock. https://www.shutterstock.com/catalog/collections/299110406 0586722847- 479dc02d89b774113d35b424fd0cb1942546c056b5128da35473 1112600200b2

Popov. (n.d.). *Continuous Glucose Monitor Blood Sugar.* *[Image].* Shutterstock. https://www.shutterstock.com/catalog/collections/299111554 7501921725- 394d65652128d41229283d3271eb767fd89932503bf8cca4371c0 f9a8fb5ec68

SewCream. (n.d.). *Woman hands making a heart shape.* *[Image].* Shutterstock. https://www.shutterstock.com/catalog/collections/299110079 8944937552- f1ee5dd034f6cdacd354720fb4f382e05da12855b05da9f6adb8d5 d2dd634690

Shutterok. (n.d.). *Multiple type of Fast food on table.* *[Image].* Shutterstock. https://www.shutterstock.com/catalog/collections/299108491 2154511009-

26738bca04598ae1d1f7b81788fa71364bf2c214c26e8783267549
803273c557

Si Janko Ferlic. (). *[Salmon with lemon]* *[Image]*. Unsplash. https://unsplash.com/photos/xgWeeJA0lUI

Silvia. (2018, May 12). *[Older women walking]* *[Image]*. Pixabay. https://pixabay.com/photos/women-girlfriends-nature-walk-3394510/

Stockcreations. (n.d.). *Heart-shaped plate of healthy heart foods.* *[Image]*. Shutterstock. https://www.shutterstock.com/catalog/collections/299109224 0123692888- d4e92ad35b89a8945256e7438097f608b7b799168e7cc84999255 5add70bebcf

Vega, T. (2018, December 9). *[Woman practicing yoga]* *[Image]*. Unsplash. https://unsplash.com/photos/F2qh3yjz6Jk

Vlasova, A. (n.d.). *Balanced nutrition concept for clean eating.* *[Image]*. Shutterstock. https://www.shutterstock.com/catalog/collections/299105094 4499680780- 265d22da2f59ff64dc430193a31a6e2bd5c32db9432aac65be5087 4f31e3e551

Made in the USA
Las Vegas, NV
30 September 2024